CHINESE PLANETARY HERBAL

DIAGNOSIS

BY

MICHAEL TIERRA C.A., O.M.D.

AND

LESLEY TIERRA C.A.

TABLE OF CONTENTS

Part I

CHINESE MEDICAL THEORY

Introduction

This booklet is a concise introduction to the theoretical principles of Traditional Chinese Holistic Herbal Diagnosis used in conjunction with the practice of Chinese herbology, acupuncture, dietetics, and related physiotherapies. The utilization of this non-medical ancient system of analysis incorporates the harmony and health of the total individual body, mind and spirit. It is the basis of development for Planetary Herbology, a system incorporating herbs, formulas and therapies from all parts of the world. It includes traditional Chinese, East Indian Ayurvedic and traditional Western herbs which are often used either separately or together in the same formula.

Basically this system of analysis differs from the Western medical approach in that it's emphasis is more energetically oriented, classifying herbs and foods according to heating-cooling or yin-yang properties. This is an approach with which I have found similar historical counterparts in traditional cultures throughout the world.

I have based this work primarily on the diagnostic principles of Traditional Chinese Medicine. This is because the Chinese have been able to preserve and continue to evolve their herbal medical system for over 5000 years, remaining today as a clear natural medical alternative for many countries of both Occidental and Oriental origin.

It is further hoped that the book will provide a theoretical foundation to the use of Planetary Herbal Formulas along with other traditional Chinese formulations and herbal treatments offered.

1

1. HERBS AS SPECIAL FOODS

Herbs can be thought of as "special foods." By so doing, we can avoid the often grave mistake of seeking for dangerously strong alternatives to our health problems, using chemical drugs often with known side effects when mild natured herbs could serve our purposes as well or better. The basic approach and understanding for the use of herbs is as special foods for specific organs and physiological processes. The three basic ways in which herbs work is 1) maintain (balance), 2) tonify and build, and 3) eliminate and detoxify. Common foods do this also but herbs work in a special way to further this process and can be of significant benefit during disease.

If herbs can be used as special foods, foods can also be used in a special therapeutic way as well. In this the two basic axioms of Hippocrates are like a motto for herbalists throughout the world, " the body heals itself" and "let your food be your medicine and your medicine your food."
Mild herbs are non-toxic, and therefore have no harmful side effects. Still, there is an underlying energetic philosophy that extends itself to include all herbs as well as foods.

The energy of herbs is traditionally described as hot, warm, neutral, cool, cold. Hot not only describes their atmospheric temperatures but the ability to generally raise body metabolism. Warm is a lesser degree of this quality. Usually, herbs that are spicy or sweet tasting are hot, warm or yang in nature. Cool or cold natured herbs are more yin and lower body temperature as well as metabolism, if it is too high. Cool or cold natured herbs tend to have bitter, sour or salty flavors. Neutral is more moderate and foodlike and has a bland flavor.
The goal is to work with, rather then against nature, following the principle of heteropathy. Yang and hot natured diseases are treated with yin, cool natured herbs and foods. Yin or cold natured diseases are treated with yang and warm natured herbs and foods. Diseases that are characterized by excess such as hypertension, toxicity and constipation are treated with more eliminative cool natured herbs. Diseases that are characterized by weakness and debility are treated by tonics. The herbalist is also able to counteract excess dampness

and fluid stagnation, relieve nervous tension and augment reproductive hormones to promote longevity and wellness.

Besides the four atmospheric energies of hot-warm-cool-cold, herbs are also classified into the five flavors and four tendencies. The five flavors describe at least part of the physiological reaction that herbs will produce based upon their taste(s). The flavors are also grouped in terms of yin and yang. The pungent and sweet flavors disperse upward and belong to yang; the salty, sour and bitter flavors flow downwards and belong to yin. The mild or bland flavor is said to leak and flow and belongs to yang.

The four tendencies of herbs are upward, outward, inward and downward. This corresponds with diseases that exhibit corresponding tendencies. Upward diseases might have symptoms of vomiting, hiccup or asthma. Outward diseases might including fever, perspiration or night-sweats. Inward diseases tend to be more chronic and more actively involve internal organic processes. Downward diseases could be diarrhea, excessive menstruation or hemorrhoids. Herbs that have a spicy flavor and lighter quality treat the surface, while herbs that have bitter, sweet, salty or sour flavors treat internally.

From this we can see how Planetary Herbology aims at treating the whole person whenever possible, not simply to eliminate a single symptom. Thus there is a more integral view of the individual as a whole uniting internal aspects including the emotions along with the immune response to external environmental influences. Diet, exercise and proper rest also plays an important role in treatment.

Although specific herbs and formulas are taken to counterbalance states often associated with disease, the Planetary herbalist, along with his or her Oriental counterpart, does not necessarily subscribe to the idea that there is a specific herb for a specific disease. What is understood is that there are some specific strategies that can be used with herbs to bring about positive organic changes. This is encompassed in the general concept of Yin and Yang.

2. CHI: THE PRINCIPLE OF UNITY

Chi is the term used by the Chinese to represent the unifying energy of all phenomena. Everything in the universe is comprised of, and defined by Chi. Yet, it can only be perceived as function rather than substance. It is the presence and quality of Chi that allows certain foods and herbs, for instance, to react favorably or adversely upon animals in general, and humans in particular, depending upon the Chi of their own native constitution.

The basic quality associated with Chi is movement, evolution and/or change. Because the nature of chi is essentially ephemeral, the knowledge of it's presence is therefore bound up with more subjective aspects of perception, such as the quality and sense of movement, odor, sound, color and form rather than the actual substance associated with these phenomena. Thus, Chi is intimately connected with the intuitive and spiritual realms although not necessarily exclusive to these levels of perception.

The great symbol of Chi to people is the sun, which is a cosmic mass that generates profound thermal energy. Any definition of chi that describes it in terms of limitation is at best, only a limited definition used for the sake of description. Chi is essentially unlimited and can be equated with concepts of the Supreme Ultimate. Various Chi's are designated, however, which is a way of describing, for instance, the effect of chi upon one's sense of vitality, exuberance, digestive capacity, growth and reproductive power. There is also the less obvious Chi of one's inherited constitution which is a predetermining power for one's general health and healing capacity throughout life.

3. YIN-YANG: ENERGY AS DUALITY

Chi, being the basic energy connecting all material and invisible phenomena, can only be perceived in terms of it's dual influences equated in terms of Yin and Yang. The more there is an imbalance between these two aspects of being, the more chi is physically experienced. It is said that energy, itself, cannot be directly perceived except beyond our sensory level of awareness and so is more akin to heightened states of religious experience described as bliss or enlightenment. Our practical experience of energy is always in terms of duality, such as Yin-cold versus Yang-hot, Yang-strong versus Yin-weak, Yin-moist versus Yang-dry and Yang-external versus Yin-internal. Thus, everything is caught up in the inescapable fact of duality.

Yin and Yang Theory is simply a way of describing the relative state of balance or imbalance of the overall individual in relation to all factors of his/her existence. Thus, diet and herbs must be adjusted according to seasonal and individual lifestyle considerations to be truly healing. During the cold seasons, it may be more appropriate to eat foods of a more substantial yang-warming nature such as cooked whole grains with a little animal protein, and cooked rather than raw vegetables and fruit. On the other hand, during the hotter climates one might use more seasonal raw fruits and vegetables.

Children, having a much higher metabolism, can tolerate a little more yin-cooling fruits than older adults whose metabolism may be lower. Similarly, a woman who is pregnant might require less Yang-heating foods and more Yin-cooling things at different stages of her pregnancy, also because of a higher yang metabolism. In all cases, whole grains as the "staff of life" and representing the balance of all parts of the life cycle of a plant and of Yin and Yang energies, should constitute the central pillar of our "daily bread." Thus, we must learn to adjust our diet and health program so that it is in harmony and balance with all external and internal emotional changes we might be experiencing.

Herbs are also classified according to Yin-Yang characteristics as they have the potential of either raising the organic metabolic function of an organ process that may be too weak or low, or lowering it if it is too high and congested. Thus, like foods, the basic energetic classification of herbs is according to their relative hot-warm-neutral-cool-cold characteristics and given to individuals to balance excessive or deficient states.

Since all people are individuals, to achieve the maximum effectiveness with herbal therapy we must learn to analyze the energetic state of the individual and his/her specific organ functions. In Traditional Chinese Medicine, the Yin-Yang Theory is applied to the state of individual organ functions, such as the " Yin of the kidney" (referring to that aspect of kidney function that relates to fluid balance and urine), or the "Yang of the kidney" (relating to the function of the adrenal glands). Because the kidneys are central to the entire theory of Chinese Medicine, they are considered the "storehouse of chi" and the "root of Yin and Yang" for the whole body. This means that the kidneys, through the complex action of adrenal medulla and cortical hormones, is able to regulate organic functions of the entire body. Thus, the kidneys are fundamental to the basic inherited constitution of the individual as a whole and the source of "inherited Chi" or "ancestral Chi." Herbs that tonify kidney Yin are demulcent-diuretics, such as asparagus root and rehmannia glutinosa, while herbs that tonify kidney Yang have warming diuretic properties, such as Juniper and dogwood berries and cinnamon.

With some organ functions, it is important to maintain a balance of Yin and Yang function. For instance, the lungs need to maintain a proper balance of moisture (Yin) and dryness (Yang), and need the Yang strength for inhalation and the Yin potential for exhalation. Therefore, there are specific treatments for the "Yang of the lungs" or the "Yin of the lungs." Herbs that increase the Yang of the lungs are Chi tonics such as ginseng, codonopsis and astragalus, and herbs that are warming and stimulating, such as anise seed, elecampane and angelica. Herbs that increase the Yin of the lungs are cooling, demulcent herbs, such as comfrey and marshmallow roots.

The heart also needs a proper balance of Yin (blood and fluids) and Yang (neurological impulse) to function properly. The yang function of the heart refers to the impulse, arterial and venous pressure while the Yin function refers to the quality and amount of blood present and the basic substance of the heart muscle. Thus, many heart problems are caused from exhaustion of heart Chi which is a Yang phenomena requiring herbs such as Ginseng, lack of heart Yin and blood, which is a Yin phenomena requiring herbs such as Chinese dang quai, congestion of Yin fluids and blood perhaps caused by a general excess of both Yang and Yin resulting in poor organ function requiring diuretic and blood moving emmenagogue herbs such as hawthorne berries and/or motherwort herb, or what is called "heart fire" which is a general condition of hyperfunction of the heart and circulation usually associated with an acidic condition of the blood requiring alterative herbs such as coptis, golden seal, and/or oregon grape root.

The liver tends to require more Yin (blood and fluids) to function properly so that it is most frequently threatened with an Excess-Yang syndrome associated with diseases of hypertension, depression and anger. Thus, herbs that are useful for the liver might be of a cool nature, such as dandelion root; tonify ying Blood and Yin, such as Chinese lycii berries; and relieving wind or spasms, such as lobelia or cramp bark. A category of warm natured herbs useful for regulating and smoothening liver Chi are carminative herbs such as fennel seed, cyperus and citrus peel. These latter herbs actually help stimulate the production and secretion of enzymes by the liver to aid digestion.

The spleen-pancreas, on the other hand, being responsible for a variety of functions associated with digestion and assimilation of food and fluids, has a basically Yang function. Therefore, the most frequent problem of the spleen-pancreas is "lack of spleen Yang," a condition associated with edema, damp swelling, poor digestion, hypoglycemia, fatigue and tiredness. Herbs that tonify Chi, such as ginseng, codonopsis and astragalus, as well as diuretics, such as atractylodes, the mushroom called poria cocos and the Western gravel root, are all good herbs to use for strengthening the spleen.

Chi and the Yin-Yang theory are the unifying theoretical basis of Traditional Chinese Medicine (TCM) and connects the individual with all aspects of being. They are not, however, always so easy to identify and determine, so that the theory, in itself, represents an essential thought process for gaining an understanding and intuitive feeling for all natural phenomena. To even begin considering things in terms of Yin and Yang is, in itself, a profound healing idea regardless of the conclusions. The accompanying chart describing Yin-Yang should be continually studied and meditated upon by any student of Chinese-Planetary herbology.

Qualities of Yin and Yang

	Yin	Yang
Tendency:	to condense	to develop
Position:	inward	outward
Structure:	space	time
Direction:	descending	ascending
Color:	dark	bright
Temperature:	cold	hot
Weight:	heavy	light
Catalyst:	water	fire
Light:	dark	light
Construction:	interior	exterior
Work:	psychological	physical
Attitude:	introspect	extrovert
Biological:	vegetable	animal
Energy:	receptive	aggressive
Nerves:	Parasympathetic	sympathetic
Tastes:	Sour-bitter-salty	spicy-sweet
Season:	Winter	Summer

Laws Governing Yin and Yang

1. All things are the differentiated apparatus of One Infinity.
2. Everything changes.
3. All antagonisms are complementary.
4. No two things are identical.
5. Every condition has its opposite.
6. Extremes always produce their opposite.
7. Whatever begins has an end.

Theorems of Yin and Yang

1. Infinity divides itself into Yin and Yang.
2. Yin and Yang result from the Infinite movement of the Universe.
3. Yin is centripetal and Yang is centrifugal; together they produce all energy and phenomena.
4. Yin attracts Yang and Yang attracts Yin.
5. Yin repels Yin and Yang repels Yang.
6. The force of attraction and repulsion between any two phenomena is proportional to the difference between their Yin-Yang constitution.
7. All things are ephemeral and changing their Yin-Yang constitution.
8. Nothing is neutral; either Yin or Yang is dominant.
9. Nothing is solely Yin or Yang; everything involves polarity.
10. Yin and Yang are relative: large Yin attracts small Yin and large Yang attracts small Yang.
11. At the extreme of manifestation, Yin produces Yang and Yang produces Yin.
12. All physical forms are Yin at the center and Yang on the surface.

4. HSU and HSIH

These terms describe the relative strength or intensity of Yin or Yang in the body. They are more subjective, measuring the quality of energy rather than the mere quantity. Hsu and Hsih (pronounced "shu and shih") represent two extremes of opposites with Hsu representing low-intensity while Hsih represents high intensity. An example of Yang-Hsih for instance, is during the final stages before death when the Yang rallies for a final jolt.

Various diseases must be treated according to Hsu and Hsih which means to interpret them according to the relative strength of Yin or Yang function. Thus, constipation is a disease that can be caused by Yang-Hsih, which means Excess and stagnation with the treatment being to purge; or it can be caused by Yang-Hsu by low nervous energy and the treatment needing tonification. Similarly, diabetes can be caused by overeating rich foods creating Yin-Hsih congestion, or chronically poor function of the pancreas, or Yin-Hsu of the pancreas.

The term "Yin Deficiency" is a condition that comes about as a result of depletion of Yin-essence with an apparent condition of Yang-Excess. Thus, there may be various paradoxical or false Yin or Yang symptoms that arise as a result of Yin or Yang Hsih or Hsu.

A depleted Hsu condition must be accompanied with tonification therapy although the primary symptoms of false-Yang must also be attended to as well. For instance, an herbal laxative for a Yang-Hsu condition might include a purgative or lubricating laxative along with tonic herbs such as dang quai and/or ginseng in order to activate the primary herbs. A treatment of inflammation or flu with echinacea in a Yang-Hsu condition might be accompanied with a lesser amount of ginseng and licorice to activate the action of the echinacea.

Paradoxically, a condition of apparent Excess such as obesity may be caused by a Hsih condition with Excess Yin requiring not only eliminative and cooling herbs, but herbs and foods that raise metabolism.

Following the concept of Hsih and Hsu, we encounter a radical diversion from Western medicine and allopathic herbal treatment which describes substances statistically according to their overall properties and indications. This means that the description of herbal properties such as a stimulant, for instance, which is intended to stimulate energy and vitality, may actually help one to relax and sleep better if one's condition is Hsu or generally depleted. This also explains why some who take panax ginseng, for instance, may experience drowsiness rather than an increase in energy as is more usual. Their basic condition may be so Hsu or depleted internally that the ginseng is too strong for them. Since ginseng is good for all kinds of deficiencies, however, one course is to begin with a much smaller Dosage to achieve the desired tonic effect.

Generally speaking, herbs are also classified according to their being Hsu and Hsih with the heavier and solid more nutritive herbs such as seeds, roots, barks being more Hsih while the more therapeutically active lighter leaves and flowers are more Hsu. Thus, the selection of appropriate herbs for individual conditions may be the use of lighter leaves, flowers and therapeutically active herbs, such as rhubarb or golden seal for Hsih conditions, while the more nutritive heavier roots and barks, such as slippery elm bark, comfrey root and rehmannia glutinosa are for Hsu conditions.

5. THE EIGHT PRINCIPLES

In studying the ancient healing systems of the planet, we find a common thread in categorizing herbs and foods according to their energetic function, their flavors, general organs and neurological pathways (called "meridians" in Chinese Acupuncture).

Chinese diagnostics, being "holistically" oriented, uses several systems of diagnosis that often overlap each other and provide a system of viewing the same problem from several different perspectives. While each system in itself may have evolved at a different time historically, this approach of using them simultaneously has become what is contemporary Traditional Chinese Medicine.

The value of the energetic classification is so obvious that one can only wonder how it could be overlooked as a factor of disease in orthodox Western medicine. In a sense, all substances can be classified as being Yin, with a hypo-metabolic effect, or Yang, with a hyper-metabolic effect. Though this may expose several areas of ambiguity in classification and treatment, the value might well be considered the essential criterion of all healing.

The Chinese approach of declining the meaning of Yin and Yang into the Eight Principles avoids the tendency for dogmatic rigidity. It allows for paradoxical symptoms which can frequently occur where, for instance, we might find hot and deficient or internal and Excess together, and thus makes the Yin and Yang imbalances more discernable.

The Chinese Eight Principles are as follows:

> Hypo-metabolic (asthenic)
> Internal (chronic diseases)
> Deficient
> Cold (low metabolism)
> Yin

Hyper-metabolic (sthenic)
External (acute diseases)
Excess
Hot (high metabolism)
Yang

Internal-External locates the depth of disease activity so we can use the appropriate approach. Examples include using sweating herbs to disperse External Heat, purgatives, cholagogues, or alteratives to relieve Internal Heat, and spicy flavored herbs such as cinnamon, ginger or cayenne for Internal or External Coldness. To this we may add herbs that relieve External and/or Internal tension and spasms called "Wind".

Deficient-Excess tells about the strength of the disease in relation to the strength of the patient. For Deficiency we would use Blood, energy, Yin or Yang tonics such as dang quai, astragalus root, asparagus root or ginseng. For Excess we would use herbs that have more active dispersing qualities such as purgatives, cholagogues, alteratives, diuretics, expectorants, or diaphoretics.

If there is "Yin Deficiency" with false heat signs and ungrounded nervous energy, we would first try to clear the heat signs before giving tonics for the Yin Deficiency lest the chosen tonic feeds the problem more than the cause. Herbs chosen for this purpose are called "clear the heat and cool blood" herbs. They include cooling herbs of more solid types, such as roots and barks with a cool, demulcent, sweetish flavor like comfrey, marshmallow root, lily of the valley root, cramp bark, figwort and Chinese herbs such as moutan peony and rehmannia glutinosa. These are chosen instead of empty energy type herbs such as leaves and flowers since we are still dealing with a deficient condition. Since there are "false Heat" signs with Yin Deficiency, we would avoid using strong warming stimulants with a spicy taste or warm-Yang energy.

If there is "Yang Deficiency" with accompanying coldness and perhaps clear fluid discharges such as clear mucus, frequent clear urination and weak digestion, we must first warm the Yang and move the Chi using internally warming stimulants, carminatives (Chi regulation) or emmenagogues.

Cold-Hot describes whether the condition is the result of a hyper-metabolic (hot) or hypo-metabolic (cold) state. Conditions not so extreme are classified as Warm, Cool or Neutral, and most people will fall under the category of warm or cool. Warm to hot may exhibit acute inflammation, fever, red face, red tongue with possible yellow and/or thick fur, faster pulse rate (over 80 beats per minute), constipation, scanty and darkish colored urine, aggressive behavior, loud voice and similar excessive conditions. For Warm to Hot conditions we would use Cool natured foods and herbs such as alteratives, heat relieving herbs that purify the blood, chologogues, laxatives, diaphoretics, cooling expectorants, cooling diuretics, antipyretics, cooling Yin tonics, and cool natured nervines.

Cold to cool will exhibit symptoms of cold extremities, preference for warmth in food, drinks and season, pale complexion, pale tongue body with clear to whitish fur, slow pulse, loose bowels, light colored urine, timid behavior, soft spokenness and a lack of motivation or drive. For this condition we use herbs that have a warm energy like warming diaphoretics, stimulants, carminatives, expectorants, nervines or antispasmodics and Yang tonics.

Yin-Yang represents a consensus of all the six preceding factors. For Deficiency of Yin there will be obvious Excess Yang symptoms, and we use Yin tonics of a cool, moist sweet flavor together with herbs that will dissipate the Excess Yang symptoms. For Deficiency of Yang, we use Yang tonics of a warm, dry, sweet or acrid flavor and herbs that will clear dampness, warm coldness, improve digestion, strengthen immunity and generally tonify Yang.

Combinations of the above syndromes include half Excess, half deficient, half Internal, half external and half cold-half hot. These kind of conditions are the most commonly encountered, the most difficult to treat and require what is called harmonization therapy using varied combinations of detoxification and tonification, cooling and warming, internal and external applied simultaneously as seems appropriate. The most commonly used formula for this kind of condition is the Chinese Minor Bupleurum Combination.

Paradoxical symptoms such as Deficiency with Heat signs mean that the nervous system is being overworked and can be called "false Yang", or if extreme, "Yin Deficiency." Excess with cold likewise means that there is an impairment of the nervous system and is called "false Yin". Excess Yin is similar to Yang Deficiency, while Excess Yang is similar to lack of Yin.

Thus, what is missing from Western medicine and the popular understanding of Western herbology is the distinction that there are warm or cool natured medicines in every therapeutic category such as nervines, diaphoretics, tonics, diuretics, and so forth. Further, similar pathologies can express themselves as being either of a Cool, Warm, Internal, External, Excess or deficient nature and require different approaches for effective treatment.

6. THE THREE HUMOURS: CHI, BLOOD AND FLUID

Chi, Blood and Fluid are essential physiological substances that form the basis for all organic function. It is not unsimilar in concept to the Ayurvedic Tridosha principle, or Three Humours, which forms the basic diagnostic method of Ayurvedic medicine. So also in Chinese medicine Chi, Blood and fluid is an essential diagnostic concept.

Chi represents that which supplies motivation, warmth and Yang action for the body. Blood is similar to that of Western medicine. Fluid describes the various fluidic substances including saliva, sweat, urine, tears, lymph and other secretions. Both Blood and Fluid are considered Yin in nature and possess the ability to nurture, moisten and lubricate. The anabolic phase of generation, growth and development as well as the catabolic phase of aging, death and disease development are involved with the dynamic interaction of Chi, Blood and fluid.

Essence denotes the essential Chi in its broadest sense sometimes referred to as the "righteous Chi", it also denotes the micro-essence or "Jing" which refers to the semen and/or reproductive capacity. Probably in its broadest and most comprehensive sense, "Essence" refers to the overall hormonal strength that regulates normal growth, metabolism and sexuality which, according to the Chinese, is stored in the kidneys-adrenals.

Diseases are understood as being involved in one or a combination of the three humours and are so denoted according to the following symptomology:
Blood disease includes circulatory problems and stagnant or extravasated blood, such as anemia, varicose veins, arteriosclerosis and hemorrhage. Extravasated blood with congealment in the capillaries, abdomen or pelvis and can give rise to a variety of symptoms including edema obesity, menstrual problems, pelvic pains and bluish or purplish discoloration. For this category, blood moving, blood regulating or blood tonic herbs are used, Blood moving herbs can be either warm or cool and are emmenagogues, blood regulating herbs are hemostatic and blood tonic herbs are nourishing.

Fluid diseases include lymphatic and general fluid metabolism and cellular metabolism which, when not properly functioning, will give rise to tumors, cysts and cancers. Water diseases involve the urinary and excretory systems. Lower symptoms include frequent urination, diarrhea, and constipation. Upper symptoms include vomiting, palpitations, tinnitus, headaches, fatigue, expectoration, salivation, rheumatic joint pains, stiffness, asthmatic breathing, cough, and thirst. Outside symptoms are edema, arthritis and sweating. The approach is to use herbs that eliminate excess fluid such as diuretics and expectorants. Certain conditions associated with Excess also require the use of purgatives as well.

Chi diseases comprise the most common disease states because Chi is the very foundation of life. Without Chi the body would be an ennervated, formless mass without life. Chinese medicine is unique in its preoccupation with Chi as the cause of disease. Chi and Blood form a polarity like Yang and Yin. Each influences the other inextricably. When there is a lack of Chi, fluid or water will accumulate so that Chi is also necessary for regulating Water disease.

Rising Chi conditions include vomiting, vertigo, headaches, and hiccups and are treated with mild purgatives. Melancholic or stagnant Chi is treated with carminatives and warming stimulants. Chi diseases are also responsible for various mental and emotional disorders. Since Chi diseases affect the nervous system, including the mind, they are among the most difficult conditions to cure.

A fourth category might be included here which encompasses food intoxication which are diseases caused from imbalanced diet and results in the accumulation of toxins. A wide variety of symptoms are caused by this problem which often is a factor in all of the above mentioned diseases. Too much or too little food can cause Excess or Deficiency conditions. Too cold or too hot can aggravate cold or hot conditions, too wet or too dry aggravates Water diseases. Foods that are extremely sweet, spicy, salty, sour or bitter can give rise to all symptoms of Blood, Water and Chi diseases.

7. THE CHINESE FIVE PHASES

The Chinese Five Phase system was perhaps first described in the medical classics, Su Wen, Ling Shu and Nan Ching, all of which are thought to have originated in the later part of the first millennium B.C.. This system of diagnosis describes the functional, dynamic relationship of internal organ systems and physiological processes. It ingeniously describes the interaction of all parts of the individual with both the internal physiological and psychological processes and the external factors such as season, climate, foods and other conditions. By so doing it shows us how an imbalance in one phase or organ process can influence an imbalance in all other facets. It is derived from and includes the Yin-Yang concept but represents a further subdivision of energetic classification into particular Organs.

With the Chinese five phase system there are many correspondences with the four elements of Graeco-European traditions, five elements of East Indian Ayurvedic medicine and the four directions of the Native North Americans. In each case, a symbolic language is used to describe a dynamic process of psycho-physiological transformation and change based upon the four directions, season, color, sound, emotions, food, organs and so forth. Certain things are said to strengthen a particular element or process while other things are considered to weaken or discharge it.

The idea is that life is a process of constant flow and change, and to inhibit that flow in any way is to give rise to disease and death. All phenomena, including herbs and foods, are contained in the five phase cycle so that various aspects can be used to execute a balance of engendering and controlling. Therefore, the system is used as another way of describing the manner in which health is maintained and disease arises from imbalances.

The correspondences of the Chinese five element cycle are as follows:

	Wood	Fire	Earth	Metal
Planet:	Jupiter	Mars	Saturn	Venus
Direction:	East	South	Center	West
Season:	Spring	Summer	Indian Summer	Autumn
Color:	Blue Green	Red	Yellow	White
Injurious Climate:	Wind	Heat	Moisture	Dryness
Yin Organ:	liver	Heart	Spleen pancreas	Lungs
Yang Organ:	Gall Bladder	Small Intestines	Stomach	Colon
Sense:	Sight	Speech	Taste	Smell
Body:	Muscles	Pulse	Flesh	Skin
Part:	Nails	Complexion	Lips	Body Hair
Orifice:	Eyes	Ears	Mouth	Nose
Fluid:	Tears	Sweat	Lymph	Mucus
Sound:	Cry	Laughter	Song	Sob
Spiritual Qualities:	Spirit	Conscience	Ideas	Instinct
Emotion:	Anger	Joy	Worry	Grief
Dynamic:	Blood	Intuition	Strength	Vitality
Governs:	Lungs	Kidney	Liver	Heart
Activity:	Seeing	Walking	Sitting	Reclining
Food Correspondences:				
Grains:	Wheat	Corn	Millet	Rice
Animal:	Chicken	Lamb	Cow	Horse
Vegetable:	Leek	Shallot	Hollyhock	Scallions
Fruits:	Plum	Apricot	Date	Peach
Better Eaten:	Sweet	Acid	Salty	Bitter
Better avoided:	Spicy	Salty	Sweet(also sour)	Sour(also bitter)

THE CHINESE FIVE PHASES

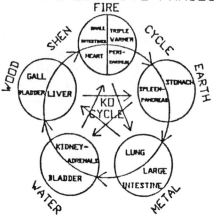

Each of the Five Phases has a dynamic inter-relationship with each other. The Shen cycle moves clockwise and is the engendering or creative movement. Thus, fire creates an ash that engenders earth; earth creates or engenders metal; metal turns into a liquid when it melts to engender fluidity; water nourishes the growth of the plant kingdom so it engenders wood and finally, wood when it burns, feeds fire.

The Ko cycle is sometimes referred to as the controlling cycle. By this, wood controls earth by pushing through soil during its growth, earth controls water by damming it, water controls fire by putting it out, fire controls metal by melting it and metal controls wood by breaking it.

Within each phase there are Yin and Yang organs that are closely related following the husband-wife law, which means to help one is to benefit the other and to harm one is to harm the other. Thus, the stomach is the husband of the spleen-pancreas; the colon is the husband of the lungs; the kidneys are the wife of the bladder, the liver is the wife of the gall bladder and the small intestine is the husband of the heart. So to treat the

20

husband-stomach is to help the process of assimilation represented by the wife-spleen-pancreas; to treat the wife-kidneys is to help the husband-bladder and so forth.

Each phase embodies a particular energy or power as follows: wood=birth, ideation, creativity, expression; fire= impulse, consciousness, spirit, mental processes; earth= centeredness, nourishment; metal= elimination, letting go, regulation and conductor of energy throughout the body; water= will power, essential power, inherited constitution, fluidity.

Thus, an imbalance of wood will cause an Excess or Deficiency in one's creativity and expressivity with the resultant feelings of frustration giving rise to anger, moodiness and depression. The individual will tend to have a shouting, angry tone of voice even in normal speech or if deficient in wood, s/he may be very timid and held in with little tendency to expression.

An imbalance in fire will cause an excess or marked lack of happy, good feelings. Thus fire or heat imbalances will influence one's ability to enjoy one's self, with an excess or marked lack of spirit. Since the heart also rules mental powers, conscience and speech, one with an imbalance of heart Chi can have mental problems, problems relating with the external world and others, a marked tendency towards psychic abilities and be either very talkative or very quiet.

An earth imbalance represents problems in assimilation of either food, drink or, on the more subtle level, ideas and concepts. There may be a lack of centeredness and grounding, a tendency to look to others for personal support, a yellowish pallor and an overly sweet manner of expression with perhaps a sing-song voice or total absence of vocal inflection.

An imbalance in metal may cause a general blockage of energy flow, giving rise to stiffness, rigidity, or an inability to let go of past occurrences. The individual may have a whining or sobbing sound to their voice, whitish palor, a tendency towards mucus, physical weakness, lung problems, sinus congestion and/or cough.

A water imbalance will be observed with inherited weaknesses, lack of will power, lack of power or strength, aching feelings in the lower back or joints and a tendency towards fatigue, dark coloration and a low, groaning or gravelly sound to the voice.

During health there will be a dynamic balance between all the Five Phases and internal physiology, but in sickness imbalance is evident between one or more of the organic cycles. This will reflect itself both physically as well as on the mental level. If wood is in excess, there will be a condition of negative influence over earth so that digestion will be effected with a tendency towards indigestion, gas, acid belching and nausea. If wood is deficient, the liver will adversely effect one's ability to gain weight, blood and lymphatic toxicity, weak digestion and infertility. If fire is over-dominant there may be symptoms of over talkativeness, tendency to inappropriate laughter and giddiness, feelings of excessive heat with redness of the face, heart and circulatory problems. Heart excess can give rise to cardio-pulmonary disease because the heart-fire over dominates the lungs-metal.

When earth is in excess there may be symptoms of bloating with gas and constipation. In Deficiency there will be weak digestion, difficulty to assimilate food, fluids or on the mental level, ideas. Earth can overdominate kidney-water aggravating urinary problems. Problems with digestion will be exaggerated with strong sweet cravings and a tendency towards mucus discharges. If this is reflected in the sinuses and lungs it would be considered a problem between earth and metal. If it is a discharge from the reproductive organs it would involve the liver and/or kidneys as well.

Since water is the essential power of all psycho-physiological functions of the body, we do not usually speak of an excess of water energy per se even though one may tend to have fluid retention. The fluid retention is governed by the earth-spleen's inability to transport and/or properly assimilate fluid. The water element embodying the overall regulation of the hormonal system by the kidney-adrenals, represents the basic ancestral Chi or inherited constitution. It is considered to be the root of Yin and Yang energy for the entire body-mind. Thus, homeostasis for the entire body-mind complex is maintained by the kidney-adrenals according to traditional Chinese theory. A Deficiency of the water phase describes basic inherited weaknesses and retarded growth patterns. Since it may also fail to properly nourish wood, there may be symptoms of body stiffness, dryness, impotence and infertility. Water's inability to control fire can give rise to an apparent excess of fire as in chronic fevers and certain heart and circulatory disorders. It's tendency in excess to overdominate fire can give rise to heart problems caused by severe edema and water retention.

A man with hypertension and a history of heart problems may demonstrate an overly aggressive behavior pattern suggesting an excess of liver-wood and his face and neck may be red with a marked tendency to party and overindulge in food and alcohol even into the late hours of the night. He may also experience occasional extreme fatigue with a craving for salt, suggesting a chronic kidney-water weakness causing the child-wood (liver) to lack guidance and the grandchild-fire (heart) to lack control. The result could be a stroke or heart failure. Treatment would be to subdue heart-fire using herbs with a bitter taste and cool energy such as oregon grape root or golden seal. (It is interesting that herbs with a bitter flavor tend to generally detoxify the body, remove or prevent parasites, clear acids from the tissues and blood and remove cholesterol, thus easing circulation.) Since the liver is said to rule the nerves, "liver-wind" which is a condition of nervousness, may need to be sedated with the use of nervines and antispasmodics such as valerian, Skullcap, and Ladies slipper. Herbs that open the liver and gall bladder, called "cholagogues", may need to be used such as thistle, artichoke leaves, vervaine or self heal. Strengthening the kidney-adrenals is more difficult, but nourishing herbs such as rehmannia glutinosa, dogwood berries and other herbs that are astringent-diuretics can be used. Also helpful is, a balanced diet, proper rest and activity with perhaps the addition of mildly salty foods such as seaweed.

Another example is a woman who complains of painful menstruation, depression, mood swings, and fluid retention especially before her cycle. She tends to crave sweets, feels spaced out and unfocused suggesting an imbalance in spleen-earth. She also has a tendency to feel unusually cold with a pale

23

complexion, suggesting a lack of Blood and Yang and a Deficiency of heart Chi. Her mood swings come and go like the wind and along with her fits of depression which may be an imbalance of liver-wood. Fluid retention can be either a sign of excess dampness or a lack of kidney Yang which would be aggravated by cold weather and over-indulgence in sweets. Over-indulgence in sweets could also lead to weakness of the water phase and might cause weakness of the kidneys, resulting in edema. Exaggerated sweet cravings can be a sign of the body's need for stronger and better quality nourishment, complex carbohydrates, protein and so forth which would be in keeping with the problem occurring at a time when blood is being discharged and lost. Treatment might be first to eliminate concentrated sweet and cold-natured foods and drinks, maintain proper protein level with the use of Japanese azuki beans cooked with kombu or wakame seaweed to help nourish the kidney-adrenals. The azuki beans also help eliminate fluid retention. Black Beans can also be used because of their ability to nourish the blood. Seaweeds provide an important source of organic calcium which will help to relieve the menstrual cramps. The addition of herbs and substances such as Gelatin and Dong quai (Angelica sinensis) to tonify and help circulate blood will help relieve the coldness and Blood Deficiency. If there is energy deficiency, ginseng can be added to tonify Yang and relieve Coldness and general deficiency. These herbs can be taken in a soup with other nourishing foods a week before one's period is due; in a similar manner the Planetary Women's Treasure formula can be taken.

The Five Phase System describes how we innately seek to maintain balance through our normal cravings and desires. Someone lacking in earth energy, for instance, may have an exceptional sweet craving. A moderate amount of balanced carbohydrates and proteins can help nourish the Deficiency while a concentrated amount of strong, sweet tasting foods can over stimulate the spleen-pancreas causing a further craving. Similarly a moderate amount of sea salt, miso, tamari and sea vegetables can help strengthen the water element while a large amount will injure and weaken it.

On an emotional level, we tend to be attracted to individuals who represent those qualities or elements in which we may be lacking. Thus, a person with a wood imbalance may have a tremendous amount of drive and find themselves emotionally drawn to one who is more laid back and lacking in personal ambition. How often have we seen couples in which one seems to always be full of joyfulness, laughter and high spirits representing an excess of fire while the other is more quiet and subdued (lacking in heart Chi)? People who tend to be sad with grief over a loss may find their feelings controlled by being with individuals who are inclined to laughter and light heartedness. We can also consider how in a relationship, when one member's energy changes over time, there may be a gradual lessening of attraction to each other leading to a separation.

The Five Phases shows us how natural harmony and health is maintained between ourselves and our outer environment. It also describes the interaction between the body and the psyche so that in a sense, there is an appropriate thought process that has a reciprocal influence upon our psycho-physiological makeup. Thought and human personality emanates from throughout our psycho-physiological processes, "in our guts" so to speak, while the brain is merely the executor. Thus, while our sweetness may be the result of an earth imbalance, our depression or aggression the result of an imbalance in wood and so forth, somehow we have an innate sense that there is something that is greater within us than a mere bunch of confused emotions and imbalanced physiological processes. It is our ability to transcend these tendencies through spiritual effort and work that must be a part of an enlightened state of spiritual detachment.

8. THE SIX STAGES OF DISEASE

The Six Stages was evolved by the Master herbalist of the Han Dynasty, Chang Chung-ching (A.D.142-220), whose famous text, Shang Han Lun, (Treatise On The Treatment of Acute Diseases Caused by Cold), is still revered, studied and practically utilized in the treatment of acute, contagious diseases. It is especially poignant to realize that this important text was written as a result of Chang's experiencing three-quarters of his family dying from a plague and the clumsy efforts of so many doctors to effectively respond to the rapidly changing character of acute diseases. The lesson is that to not be able to respond and alter treatment appropriately during an acute disease attack can prove to have fatal consequences.

It must be kept in mind that a disease does not necessarily have to follow the sequence described in the Six Stages but can begin at any of the three Yang stages and proceed to any of the others.

The Six stages are:

1. **Greater Yang (Tai Yang):** this stage occurs when an External disease first attacks the body's defenses. The characteristics are chills, fevers, stiffness and headache. The symptoms are often described as shivers "up and down the spine" which describes the Chinese bladder meridian that traverses along the spinal column of the back, and the Small Intestine meridian that goes along the outer arms to the upper back and shoulders. Such vulnerability to external evils will not occur if one is not already in a weakened state and one's pores (ruled by the nerve Chi that controls their opening and closing) are not able to sufficiently ward off cold and damp conditions. If we give purgatives during this stage we weaken the body from within and allow the invading external pathogens to penetrate deeper. Therefore, diaphoretic, sweating therapy is indicated.

2. **Lesser Yang (Hsiao Yang):** this stage is characteristic of more commonly found chronic diseases in which there is literally a combination of Excess and Deficiency, Cold and Heat, Internal and External. It is very characteristic of diseases

such as malaria and typhoid fevers that show alternating heat and chills, and a cyclic recurrence of symptoms indicating that the disease is at the level of the lesser Yang. In this state it more deeply involves the nervous system which is ruled by the wood element (liver and gall bladder). For this reason, the gall bladder and triple warmer meridians are considered theoretically to be the next layer below the surface (Tai Yang) layer. Harmonizing therapy is indicated.

3. Sunlight Yang (Yang Ming): this stage is always characterized by feelings of extreme heat, abdominal discomfort, constipation and unlike the previous two stages, no chills. Purgatives and/or diaphoretics are indicated here. First we would give Herbal Uprising to promote sweating and then follow with Triphala to clear stomach and bowel congestion.

4. Greater Yin (Tai Yin): this first Yin stage has signs of chills and distended abdomen with occasional pain. It is associated with the kidney and heart meridians. Internal warming therapy is given using warm stimulants with tonics.

5. Lesser Yin (Hsiao Yin): the second stage exhibits a weak pulse, anxiety, drowsiness, diarrhea, chills and cold extremities. It is associated with the spleen and lungs. Internal warming and tonics are used.

6. Absolute Yin (Chueh Yin): the last Yin stage is indicated by thirst, difficult urination and physical collapse. It is associated with the pericardium and liver. Internal warming and tonics are used.

The three Yin stages of disease are describing a further worsening of symptoms with associated weakness and coldness. All three stages require warm tonification therapies using Yang tonics to support the bodies' life force such as Tai Chi given in tea, Trikatu, and Herbal Warmth ("Su Ni Tang"). One method I have used is to give slippery elm gruel, made by adding warm water, ginseng tea or a tea of Tai Chi pills to slippery elm powder until a cereal-like consistency is achieved. This is then fed to weakened patients and is very strengthening.

It must be kept in mind that a disease does not necessarily have to follow the sequence described in the six stages, but can begin at any of the three Yang stages and proceed to any of the others.

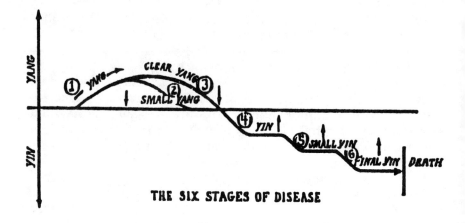

THE SIX STAGES OF DISEASE

9. EIGHT METHODS OF HERBAL TREATMENT

Chinese medicine encompasses eight therapeutic methods of treatment: sweating, vomiting, purging, harmonizing, warming, removing, supplementing and reducing.

Sweating therapy is only used for External oriented diseases and is further differentiated into External Cold or External Hot, External Deficient and External Excess. The major indication for sweating therapy is chills and fever; whereas contraindications include a severe loss of bodily fluids from vomiting and diarrhea.

Vomiting therapy is used for food poisoning, mucus accumulation causing lung congestion, abdominal pain, and so forth.

It is not used by many for the treatment of excess mucus problems, although it can be. There are usually other less drastic methods that can be followed with equal or greater effectiveness. In any case, unless one is properly trained in the approach it is safest not to attempt it for this purpose.

Vomiting is the most important method for treating food and narcotic poisoning. For this purpose, it is simplest and most effective to use syrup of Ipecac, an herbal substance that is available from most pharmacies.

Vomiting should never be done to counteract caustic poisons such as swallowing lye or various other petroleum or chemical poisons. Rather, the approach should be to dilute the poisonous substance with a protecting demulcent substance such as licorice tea, marshmallow root or slippery elm gruel. A doctor should be contacted if at all possible.

Purging therapy is indicated for elimination of toxins through the colon. Purgatives are used for Excess conformation with gastric and intestinal pains, constipation, dry stools and extravasated blood in the lower abdomen giving rise to gynecological pains and disorders. There are two types of purgatives: one is bitter and cool while the other is warm. There are also water-expelling purgatives called drastics used for Excess conformation diseases associated with fluid accumulation under the heart, sweating and asthma. Purgatives are also used to expel worms often in combination with anthelmintics.

Contraindications include all surface conformation diseases since purgatives can drive the external disease inward, also for half External and half Internal conditions requiring harmonizing therapy, and individuals with loss of fluids and associated constipation, delicate health and/or lack of vitality. They should be used with caution during menstruation, pregnancy and the postpartum period.

Harmonizing therapy is used for lesser Yang diseases involving the liver, gall bladder or stomach. It is the most commonly used herbal therapy for restoring general balance. It is given for diseases of a polarized half and half conformation.

Indications for harmonizing treatment are: 1.) liver and gall bladder diseases with intermittent fever, heart, chest pains, and nausea; 2.) Hot diseases associated with malaria, thirst and nausea; 3.) women suffering from premenstrual syndrome with elevated temperature, swelling of the abdomen, pains in the lower abdomen, mood swings and oppressed feeling in the chest.

Warming therapy uses warm stimulants to treat Cold conditions. It supplements and strengthens Yang Chi, thus it is used for restoring loss of vitality. It is useful for coldness, vomiting, abdominal pain, weak pulse, and a general cold, weak conformation.

Coldness occurs in individuals with a loss of Yang causing digestive weakness, loose stools, clear urine, weakness of body and spirit, cold extremities, poor appetite, abdominal distension and stomach pains.

Many contra-indications exist. Warming therapy should not be used with the following: 1.) those with Internal Excess and Heat with false External Cold signs; 2.) anyone with

Internal Yin Deficiency with associated spitting of blood and blood in the stools; 3.) those with fever and diarrhea, loss of energy, thin and dark face, dry skin; and 4.) those with Yin Deficiency with a black tongue and dry throat.

Removing therapy refers to alterative, blood purifying herbs which can be used to detoxify the body, remove fever and destroy pathogens without depleting body fluids and thus, weakening Essence Chi. There are three subtypes: Essence type (Chi fen), Solid type (Ying fen), and Blood type (Hsieh fen).

For Essence fever there are no chills, severe high temperature, sweating, thirst, yellow-coated, dry tongue, and a large, fast pulse. Bitter, cold clearing herbs are used such as coptis and goldenseal. A fast pulse with reddish-brown tongue is a solid fever conformation and requires fire removing, antibiotic herbs.

Blood fever also has a reddish-brown tongue, with anxiety, delirium, spitting of blood and nosebleeds. This type of fever requires Blood cooling and Heat eliminating therapy. Herbs such as rhinoceros horn, uncooked rehmannia and scrophularia are used.

Removing method is contraindicated for individuals with delicate health, cold extremities, soft stools, diarrhea, anxiety caused by a loss of blood, and those weakened by extreme physical depletion or having a severe loss of energy causing fever and weak fever.

Supplementing or tonification therapy is indicated for individuals in need of nutritional supplementation. Generally, ginseng and ginseng type herbs are considered. In Western herbology stomach bitters, helping to restore digestive fire for better assimilation, are used but only in small amounts before meals (a teaspoon or so).

Chi supplementation is given for those with fatigue, malaise, shallow breath, soft spoken voice, sub-clinical fever, involuntary sweating, weak pulse or prolapsed internal organs. Blood supplementation is for those with weak blood, paleness, tinnitus, excessive stomach acid, palpitations in the chest, and in women, menstrual irregularities and/or extravasated blood.

Yin supplementation is for those who are emaciated and weak with excessive thirst. Palpitations, insomnia, night sweats, nocturnal emission, coughing and spitting of blood are signs of Yin Deficiency. Yang supplementation is used for those with coldness, impotency, weakness, chills in the lower body, difficulty in walking, lower abdominal pain, problems with defecation, frequent urination and Deficiency asthma.

Reducing therapy is used to reduce blocked Chi, Blood and sputum, abnormal swelling, obesity, Tumors, ulcers and extravasated blood. Reducing method can resemble purgation, but in this approach the strategy is slower with the disease gradually disappearing.

Contraindications for the reducing method include weakness of Chi with abdominal distension; low grade fever, thirst, loss of appetite, diarrhea, weak digestion, and gynecological problems with loss of blood and amenorrhea.

Often combined methods are used such as the following:

Sweating and purging are used when chills, fever, headaches and stiffness are associated with constipation. The rule is first sweat, then purge.

Warming and removing are used when there are upper or lower chills or fever following infectious diseases. Warming herbs are combined with removing herbs to offset side effects and prevent loss of vitality.

Attacking and supplementing are used when the disease exhibits signs of both weakness and Excess congestion. If one gives only supplements the disease might not be uprooted; if one gives only purging, further prostration could occur. In these cases a combination of ginseng and similar tonics can be given along with purgatives.

TREATMENT PRINCIPLES

1. Supplement weakness before purging and eliminating. This is done to protect the righteous energy from degenerating.

2. Treat External diseases first before treating extravasated blood.

3. Treat the outer stem before treating the root. Treat External diseases before working on Internal weaknesses. In most even the application of cool natured, antibiotic herbs can be given to help resolve inflammatory conditions even in those who are weak and Deficient. About three days to one week can be followed in this approach. If this doesn't work, then the treatment principle should be reversed. Some formulas, such as cinnamon and ginseng can treat both inside and outside conformations at the same time.

4. Always treat cautiously at first to be sure that the condition is one of either Excess or Deficiency, Hot or Cold. Preferably begin treating as if it were a Deficient disease so as not to aggravate the illness.

5. If during the course of treating an Internal chronic disease the patient develops an acute condition, treatment for the chronic condition should be suspended for treatment of the acute.

6. Most often an appropriate herbal treatment will exhibit its positive effects within three days, in which case it should be continued. If no improvement is noted, it may, however, still be the right treatment and it should be continued anyway. Even so, called "healing crises" syndromes will occur at which time treatment may be temporarily suspended or dosage lowered for a time. A healing crisis is always accompanied by concomitant signs of improvement. It is also characterized by a shortened retracing of earlier disease syndromes.

Part II

INTRODUCTION:
DIAGNOSIS AND TREATMENT

The treatment of disease by Chinese Medicine is based on seeing the relationship of a symptom to the whole body. In this way the various signs and symptoms experienced by an individual interrelate to form a pattern of disharmony. It is this pattern then, which is treated, rather than the individual symptom. Chinese medicine is thus holistic, based on the idea that no single part can be understood except in its relation to the whole.

The causes of disease explained here are not by any means all-inclusive; there are further causes recognized by Chinese medicine. Part II, continuing from the principles in Part I, gives several causes of disease which build on one another to form the basic patterns of disharmony manifesting in the body.

In Part III the herbal categories appropriate for treating each pattern of disharmony is given. These are based on the Chinese Pharmacopeia's organization of herbs and on the Pharmacopeia outlined in <u>Planetary Herbology</u> by Michael Tierra. The corresponding Planetary formulas are also applied to these patterns so a further understanding of using the Planetary formulas is achieved. Foods and individual herbs are then included so one can creatively put together an individual plan if desired.

10. TRADITIONAL CHINESE AND WESTERN PHYSIOLOGY:
A Comparative View

Chinese Traditional Medicine developed simultaneously with early Taoist religious teachings. These teachings had their roots in nature, equating the "Tao" with the "Way" or "flow" of natural processes. Rather then establishing a religion based upon the concept of "God" or "the Great Spirit" as did later religions, they sought a direct experience of the Supreme Ultimate through close observation and harmony with inner and outer nature.

Thus, like the Native Americans for instance, Taoists perceive the Great Spirit as part of nature. They sought personal harmony with the seasons, plants, animals, things organic and inorganic as well as celestial influences of the stars and planets as the highest achievement of life. Being process oriented rather than goal oriented as are other religions, Taoist philosophy is represented by the I Ching or Taoist Book of Divination, the teachings of the Yellow Emperor, which is still the foundation of traditional acupuncture and Chinese medicine, and the great philosophers, Lao Tzu and Chuang Tsu. Taoists metaphorically compared water to the Tao, "The highest good is like water. Water gives life to the ten thousand things and does not strive. It flows in places men reject and so is like the Tao." (Tao Te Ching translated by Gia-Fu Feng and Jane English).

Even though the inevitable cycle of birth-growth-decay and death of the physical body was assumed, disease and discord was generally viewed as being in a state of personal disharmony with the Tao of one's life. Eventually, Taoists came to view the possibility of spiritual, and in a sense, even physical immortality as a possibility for one who lived according to the Tao. From this came the concept of the "immortals" which included Lao Tzu and other Taoist masters who eventually have come to be worshipped as models by Taoist followers.

As part of the nature religion of Taoism, dietary and herbal medicine was first practiced and espoused by Taoist priests, much as the Vedic and Egyptian priests of ancient times took charge of the evolution and practice of medicine. Herbs, according to the modern master Stephen T. Chang, are the "forgotten foods" which, when appropriately included in one's regular diet, can impart strength and protection to the inner, psycho-physiological life forces.

There being taboos against violating the spirit of a deceased through dissection, early Taoist physiology evolved from more intuitive approaches. Being based upon empirical observation and experience, Taoists dedicated themselves to sharpening their abilities to directly perceive energetic imbalances through the four diagnosis of looking, listening, smelling and palpating. Besides diagnosing disease, these same capacities were the basis for evaluating and classifying the therapeutic efficacy of wild plants and other treatment modalities. From this the concept of yin-yang, the five elements and 12 organs evolved.

These organs included not only their physical locations and appearances, but their dynamic actions and spheres of influence throughout the body-mind process. In view of the more specialized and mechanical anatomical description of contemporary Western medicine, the traditional understanding of Traditional Chinese Medicine, while using modern anatomical terms, can be misleading.

Further, there are at least two organic systems described as fixed entities which may have no specific location in the physical body. These are the Triple Warmer and the Circulation/Sex or what is known today as the Pericardium. The Triple Warmer seems to indicate the relationship of all the physiological parts of the upper, middle and lower parts of the body while the Circulation/Sex or Pericardium has very specific psychological indications which seem to correlate to our innate ability to relate to ourselves and others.

It is, however, possible to at least partially describe the meanings and functions of the 12 dynamic organic processes in terms of contemporary physiology. By so doing, one may have a deeper understanding and appreciation for the profound wisdom of Traditional Chinese Medicine, its diagnostic methods and treatment principles.

Following are a few examples of these as I and a few others have come to understand them:

Chi -- Perhaps the single most important concept of Traditional Chinese medicine is that of "Chi" as the pervasive motivating force of life energy both within and outside of the body. The origin of Chi is from the cosmos. Life is the ability to embrace it and use Chi energy as the fundamental aspect of beingness. On a more narrow scale, Chi can be considered the equivalent to biological nervous energy.

Meridians -- The pathways along which Chi passes and flows, these are undoubtedly both gross and subtle neurological connections.

Yang -- Yang Chi includes the outgoing masculine or motivating force as well as the body's capacity to generate and maintain warmth. It can be equated with hyper-metabolic qualities which effect all organic processes, including warmth, libido and appetite. Its normal manifestation is comparable to our concept of zest for life. In pathological excess it is synonymous with stagnation, congestion and excess heat.

Yin -- The polar opposite of Yang in terms of it being more in-going and receptive, Yin Chi is more receptive and fluidic and equated with hypo-metabolic qualities and conditions. Physiologically it represents innate capacity or substance. Thus, a lack of Yin can manifest as a lack of Chi because there is then an innate injury of an organ, nerve or other receptor that does not allow for the utilization or circulation Chi or Yang energy.

Blood -- Blood, being fluidic, is a part of Yin Chi.

Essence -- This is inherited potential which supplies nourishment for growth and maturation. In deficiency, it can also refer to that part of our being which is wasted or depleted as a part of living.

Wind -- Besides its cosmic meaning, Wind in the body, wind usually refers to a neurological response of either an external or internal stimulus. Typical neurological conditions of spasms, nervousness, twitches, numbness and convulsions are a manifestation of Wind as well as the general spread of acute disease. Wind is said to emanate from the Liver and Gallbladder which suggests that in some way these organs are responsible in significant measure for the above conditions.

Cold -- A condition of hypo-metabolic function.

<u>Heat</u> -- A condition of hyper-metabolic function, in extreme conditions it can be classed as fire which describes an inflammatory process.

<u>Damp</u> -- A condition of fluid excess characterized by fluidic discharges or edema. Damp Cold refers to more alkaline hypo-metablic excess, while Damp Heat refers to the accumulation of more acidic or inflammatory conditions.

<u>Dryness</u> -- A general lack of fluids, moisture or essence.

<u>Heart</u> -- This organ process refers to the specific organ of the Heart from which Chinese medicine states, all heat emanates. It also refers to the mind and psychological aspect of consciousness and is our outgoing capacity to relate to the outside world. Thus Chinese medicine equates the Heart with speech and consciousness. Problems involving consciousness, speech, delirium and forgetfulness for instance, are treated through the Heart. Besides the physiological Heart, many aspects associated with the thyroid gland are indicated in the concept of Heart Chi.

<u>Lungs</u> -- Besides the organs themselves, the concept of the Lungs in Chinese medicine receive, circulate and eliminate energy. Thus the Chinese Lungs extend themselves to the skin and body hair.

<u>Kidneys</u> -- The source of inherited constitutional strength and potential, the Kidneys are the most important and profound organ concept in Traditional Chinese Medicine. While it most certainly refers to the urinary organs, its deeper significance is better understood as the endocrine glands, most especially the adrenals. Kidney Yin refers to the more cooling, cortical secretions of the adrenal cortex, while Kidney Yang is the more stimulating adrenaline secretions of the adrenal medulla. Since traditional wisdom states that the inherited potential is stored in the Kidneys, it governs the process of aging. Further, the deeper energies of Kidney Chi as such cannot be acquired from food, air and water; it can only be consumed or preserved. Taoists believe that through Chi Gong or combined breathing

and concentration exercises, Kidney Chi might be acquired or optimized.

Spleen -- The second most profound concept in Chinese medicine, the Spleen is the source of acquired chi. It is through the Spleen that the energy of food, air and water is assimilated at its deepest level and utilized. Certainly the Western concept of the spleen is vastly more limited then that of the Chinese. Spleen Chi includes the deeper aspects of assimilation in the Small Intestine as well as the functions of the Pancreas. Thus, like the other organs, the concept of the Spleen is to be considered as a comprehensive function of many systems and organs, especially those associated with digestion and assimilation. In one recent report (*), research on the cellular, subcellular and molecular level closely relates the function of the traditional Chinese concept of the Spleen to the mitochondria. Mitochondria exist in all tissues and cells and are considered as the base of ATP production and the motive power of the cells. This equates with the traditional Chinese concept of the Spleen as the origin of vital energy and blood production and its being responsible for the postnatal growth of the human body.

Liver -- The Western concept of the Liver is certainly an area of vast domain and influence already. It is no surprise that the Chinese concept generally includes all the known Western physiological concepts and further psychological aspects as well. The traditional Chinese Liver seems to refer to its ability to generally detoxify the blood, store and release glycogen as needed, regulate vital digestive secretions and process hormones and other neuro-transmitting secretions. Thus the Liver becomes the third most important concept of Traditional Chinese medicine since it effects such a wide range of functions.

Pericardium -- This was described previously and generally seems to be an extension of the function of the Heart. Sometimes it is called the Heart-Protector because it is an indirect way to treat the heart with acupuncture and herbs.

Small Intestine -- As with most of the Yang organs, the Small Intestine primarily refers to its immediate sphere of influence in terms of digestion. It does, however, extend itself to include urinary or bladder infections. The idea possibly refers to infections generally as a condition of malabsorption. Thus, if the Small Intestine is unable to "separate the pure from the impure", as it is stated in the traditional literature, that which is part of the impure pollutes the blood and instead of being discharged through the Small Intestine to the Large Intestine, it is eliminated through the urinary tract, causing infections.

Large Intestine -- This almost entirely refers to the function of the colon. What is suggested here is that the colon is primarily responsible for the elimination of pathogenic Heat or inflammation in the body and that constipation is a strong indication of pathogenic Heat. If there is no constipation, then one can choose to discharge Heat or inflammatory processes by the use of cholagogues or herbs that stimulate bile secretion through the Liver-Gallbladder.

Gallbladder -- Generally referring to the conditions associated with the specific organ Western concept of Gallbladder, it does insinuate a greater meaning when we consider its association with the concept of Wind, a Yang phenomena originating in the Liver. Thus the Gallbladder in Traditional Chinese Medicine seems, for better or worse, to refer to the very essence of the bodies' mechanism of appropriate tension or spasm which extends itself to a wide sphere of influence and pathogenic conditions including neck and mental tension, migraine and other tension headaches, stroke and paralysis together with a wide variety of neurological disorders. Since it is directly treated with both antispasmodic and chologogue herbs, it is, like the Liver, associated with blood toxicity. What we can understand from the Traditional Chinese concept is that the Gallbladder, with its ability to retain bile, is the essence of appropriate tension in the body which makes it responsible for courage and decision making.

Urinary Bladder -- Besides referring to the specific Western anatomical organ, it is also the Yang counterpart of the Kidneys. Thus, at least in its meridian pathway which is the longest in the body, it is responsible for communicating and transporting the energy of the Kidneys to the brain.

Triple Warmer -- This is discussed previously and seems to be the most theoretical organ process of Traditional Chinese Medicine at least in terms of current understanding. Some have understood it as the Western physiological function of the Hypothalamus. Most recently, Kikko Matsumoto compared it to the connective tissue of the body.

(*) "An Exploration of the Nature of "Spleen" in Traditional Chinese Medicine on a Subcellular Level: A Study on the Gastric Mucosal Ultrastructure of 51 Cases" by Liu Youzhang, Guangzhou College of TCM. Published in Traditional Chinese Medicine Digest Vol. 11 Nos. 3 and 4.

II. <u>PERNICIOUS INFLUENCES</u>

Just as we experience weather in our external environment, we can feel it inside our bodies also. When normal environmental forces become excessive or occur unseasonably, they may invade the body and cause disease. However, an imbalance among the Organs internally can also lead to symptoms similar to those of an externally caused illness. In either case, both are based on symptoms which correspond to the Pernicious Influences and these manifest as climatic conditions in the body.

The six Pernicious Influences are Wind, Cold, Fire or Heat, Dampness, Dryness and Summer Heat. When the body is weakened by an imbalance, a climatic phenomenon can invade and then become an external Pernicious Influence. Illnesses generated in this way usually come on with no warning and they usually accompany sudden acute illnesses. They are characterized by aversion toward the particular influence (such as fear of cold, dislike of wind), fever, chills, body aches and general malaise.

When a Pernicious Influence arises internally, it is called an internal Pernicious Influence. In this case, the body manifests similar signs and symptoms with one important difference, the illness does not usually come on suddenly, and usually there are no fever or chills. It is often related to chronic illnesses. All Pernicious Influences, however, reflect the climatic condition and are treated accordingly.

The easiest way to understand the Pernicious Influences is to think of how their counterparts in weather manifest. For instance, wind moves things, changes direction, is fickle and alternates intensity. Water is damp and heavy, sinks to a lower level and slows things down, such as traffic. Coldness contracts like ice, and causes us to curl up by a cozy fire. Therefore, just as our environments can be windy, damp or cold, our bodies can be these ways also.

The following descriptions of each Influence include the possible signs and ways a given Pernicious Influence can manifest. Both the external and internal aspects are discussed. Three or more signs under a given category need manifest to indicate the existence of that Influence. Often, two or more Pernicious Influences appear together, such as damp-heat, damp-cold, wind-cold or wind-damp. In these cases all the Influences involved are treated.

Wind

In the body Wind has very similar qualities to the wind in weather. Essentially, it is movement and can manifest as follows:

Internal:

-numbness of limbs
-deviations, paralysis
-comes and goes fast
-convulsion
-signs change locations
-various signs appear in succession
-tetany
-tendency toward movement and change

-itching
-spasms
-floating pulse
-moving pain
-tremors

External:

-any of the above combined with sudden onset, fear of drafts

Cold

Coldness tends to congeal and contract, like ice. It will cause a person to hunch over or curl up in order to minimize body surface and maintain inner warmth. Also, with lack of heat, activity in all forms slows down.

Internal:

-feeling of coldness
-underactivity
-aversion to cold
-craves warmth
-pale moist tongue, white coat
-slow or tight and deep pulse
-lack in circulation of Chi and Blood
-pale, frigid appearance
-achy pain in joints and flesh
-clear discharges (urine, nasal, etc.)
-tendency toward stagnation and contraction

-no thirst
-no sweating
-diarrhea
-slowness
-sleeps alot

External:

the above plus:

-sudden onset
-mild fever
-little sweating

-fear of cold
-body aches
-chills

Heat

    Heat causes extreme activity in the body with a tendency to rise up and out, like the heat from a fire. When it does this, it often moves other things with it, like blood, or the tongue (speech), and so forth.

Internal:

-constipation
-thirst
-dark yellow or red urine
-craves cold
-bloody nose
-yellow mucus, stools or urine
-delirium, confused speech
-blood in any discharges
-yellow coated tongue, red tongue body
-sticky, thick and hot-feeling excretions

-red face, eyes
-dislikes heat
-scanty urination
-hemorrhaging
-irritability
-fast pulse
-tends to rise

External:

the above plus:

- high fever
- thirst
- carbuncles
- red skin eruptions
- sore, swollen throat

- sweating
- headaches
- boils
- slight chills

Note: Excess Heat can exhaust the Yin resulting in dry signs and possibly the   stirring up of Wind.

Damp

In the body dampness is like rain, it is wet, heavy, congesting and stagnating.

Internal:

- slippery or soggy pulse
- thick greasy tongue moss
- sticky sweetish taste
- no desire to drink
- feeling of fullness

- slow pulse
- nausea
- leukorrhea
- watery stool
- lassitude

- tendency toward heaviness and turbidity
- lack of appetite and sensation of taste
- heavy, stiff or sore joints
- distention or soreness in chest, head, flank or abdomen
- oozing ulcers and abscesses
- heavy diarrhea or vaginal discharge
- skin eruptions containing fluids
- copious, turbid, cloudy or sticky excretions and
  secretions
- tendency toward viscosity and stagnation

External:

- any of the above plus acute onset, low fever

Dryness

Dryness is the lack of moisture and fluids, like a desert.

Internal:

-dehydration
-dry, rough, chapped or cracked
-Yin fluids consumed
-unusual thirst
-dry stools
-dry skin
-dry tongue
-dry cough

External:

-the above plus dry and sore throat, acute onset

Summer Heat

This is a more intense Heat condition which includes Heat signs plus:

-delirium
-shortness of breath
-restlessness
-depletion of fluids
-sudden high fever
-coma
-heat stroke
-disturbed mind
-exhaustion
-profuse sweating

Phlegm

Another factor which should be included here is called Phlegm. It is essentially an extension of dampness in a stagnated or congested state. Thus, when the water in the body becomes stagnant, it transforms into Phlegm. Phlegm is both the result of dysfunction and the cause of further dysfunction.

-numbness in limbs   -slippery pulse
-greasy thick tongue moss   -tremors
-convulsions   -delirium
-sudden collapse   -muddled thought
-tends toward obstruction   -paralysis
-soft mobile -swellings, lumps or tumors

      Overall, if Phlegm collects in any of the following areas it will have the subsequent signs of Phlegm obstructing the:
      Lungs: cough, asthma, mucus
      Heart: coma, rattle in the throat
      Meridians: hemiplegia, deviation of
                 eyes and mouth, numbness of
                 limbs
      Subcutaneous layers: soft, movable nodules

12. DIFFERENTIATION OF SYNDROMES

This diagnostic category encompasses the fundamental properties of the body. It is these which sustain the normal vital activities. They include Chi, Yang, Blood, Yin and Essence. The qualities of each of these properties is:

Chi

-energy -activity
-the motivator of
bodily functions

Yang

-Chi plus heat

Blood

-blood in the body

Yin

-Blood plus all
other bodily fluids

Essence

-maturation, growth and development
-suppleness of bones
-fertility
-supportive and nutritive

-semen

Yin and Yang in the body are fundamental properties with the qualities just given. Yet, another use of the terms Yin and Yang is often made which labels a person as being "too Yin or too Yang". Using the terms in this way is a macrobiotic approach which actually refers to the state of Yin as being a condition of Deficiency and Yang a condition of Excess. This is different than the fundamental properties in the body where Yin encompasses bodily fluids and substance and Yang is Chi with Heat. Therefore, when it is said that a person has too much Yin or Yang in the body then what is meant is that s/he has an overabundance of Fluids or Heat in the body.

Now when a person is labeled as "too Yin or Yang" what is meant is that s/he is in a state of Deficiency or Excess. For instance, when a person is labeled as "too Yin" s/he is frequently thin, emaciated and showing heat signs. In this case calling this person "too Yin" is really saying that s/he is in a state of Deficiency. Whereas in terms of Yin in the body, this person is actually experiencing a lack of Yin or bodily substance and Fluids, resulting in emaciation and heat signs. Likewise, in terms of the fundamental properties of the body if it is said that a person has too much Yin, then this person exhibits signs of too much substance and Fluids, as in obesity or edema.

It is important to distinguish between these two uses of the terms Yin and Yang and to aid this process, Yin and Yang in capitals refers to the fundamental substances of Yin and Yang, whereas Yin and Yang in lower case refers to the states of Deficiency and Excess.

The various ways that the fundamental substances manifest in the body are detailed in the following.

Deficient Chi

When Chi is deficient, the primary energy is weakened, resulting in reduced functions such as:

-low, soft voice   -dislike of movement
-spontaneous sweating   -pale tongue material
-little desire to speak   -lack of appetite
-general weakness or lethargy
-shallow respiration   -empty, frail or weak pulse
-prolapse ("collapsed Chi")
-pale, bright face that is puffy or bloated
-early periods, excessive bleeding

Deficient Yang

A more severe case of Deficient Chi, Deficient Yang also includes lack of body heat, thus resulting in coldness.

49

Deficient Chi signs plus:

- cold limbs   -aversion to cold
- slow pulse   -puffy tongue
- impotence
- watery stools with undigested food in them

Stagnant Chi

This is Chi which is 'stuck' or moves improperly.

- soft palpable lumps
- darkish or purplish tongue
- wiry or tight pulse
- rebellious Chi (Chi goes in the wrong direction such as nausea or vomiting)
- distension, soreness and pain, both of which
  change in severity and location

Deficient Blood

When Blood is insufficient in the body it will manifest in these ways:

- thin, emaciated body   -numb limbs
- weak tremors in limbs   -dizziness
- dry skin or hair   -scanty menses
- pale tongue material   -thin pulse
- lusterless, pale face and lips
- spots in visual field, impaired vision

Deficient Yin

When all bodily fluids are insufficient, then dryness and heat manifest since the Yin Fluids are not lubricating as necessary.

Deficient Blood signs plus:

-agitated manner
-warm palms and soles
-insomnia
-red tongue material

-red cheeks
-rapid, thin pulse
-night sweats
-thirst

Congealed Blood

When Blood gets 'stuck' it can manifest as:

-fixed and stabbing pain
-hard, immobile masses
-choppy pulse
-clots of a dark, purple tinge
-swelling of organs
-lumps
-dark purple tongue material with red spots

-tremors
-dark complexion
-frequent hemorrhages
-tumors
-cysts

Hot Blood

When too much heat enters the Blood, it causes excessive movement which manifests as:

-bleeding
-excessive menses
-bloody nose
-delirium
-rapid pulse
-blood in sputum, vomitus, urine or stool

-red skin eruptions
-irritability
-thirst
-scarlet tongue
-hemorrhage

51

Deficient Chi and Blood

This category includes combined signs of the two individual categories of Deficient Chi and Deficient Blood.

Deficient Yin and Yang

This category combines signs from the two individual categories of Deficient Yin and Deficient Yang.

Excess Yin

This is a general condition of Damp signs as there is too much fluid in the body. (see Dampness under: Pernicious Influences.)

Excess Yang

This is a general condition of Heat signs since there is too much Chi and Heat present. (See Heat under: I Pernicious Influences.)

Deficiency of Essence

-improper maturation
-inability to reproduce
-brittle bones

-sexual dysfunction
-premature aging

13. DIFFERENTIATION OF ORGANS

The concept of the Organs in Chinese medicine is radically different from that of contemporary Western medicine. Understanding this difference is very important because the physiology and pathology of the Organs is fundamental to the understanding and treatment of disease.

Although many of the terms for the Organs are similar to Western names, they do not refer to the specific tissue. Instead, they are complexes of closely related functions. In fact, one particular Organ, the Triple Warmer, has no anatomical substrate. These are semi-abstract concepts which are based on clinical observations over hundreds of years rather than surgical discoveries. Thus, it is the outward manifestations of the complexes that are focused upon as the signs of the Organs.

The Organs are divided into two principle groups: the Yin (Inner) and Yang (Outer) Organs. The Yin Organs are the core of the entire system and are said to "store and not drain", meaning that their functions are directed toward sustaining homeostasis, both physically and mentally. The Yang Organs are said to "drain and not store", referring to their role in the transformation and disposal of food and waste. There are also two extraordinary organs, the Brain and the Uterus. These are dealt with separately.

As described in Part I under the Five Phases, each organ has a corresponding taste, color, emotion, season and so forth. Refer back to that section for review. The following lists each Organ complex with its individual signs and symptoms. Remember, for an organ to be involved in an imbalance, there must be three or more signs of that organ manifesting.

YIN ORGANS

The Yin organs sustain physical and mental balance in the body. They perform the vital functions.

Heart

-stores shen (spirit)   -opens to the tongue
-heart's brilliance manifests in the face
-controls the blood, vessels and circulation
-houses the mind: spirit, consciousness, memory,
 thinking and sleep

-palpitations   -hysteria
-forgetfulness   -insanity
-excessive dreaming   -delirium
-irrational behavior

Lungs

-rules skin and body hair   -opens to the nose
-dominates air (rules Chi)
-dispersing function   -Chi descends
-residence of protective Chi (wei Chi)
-regulates water passages and promotes water
 metabolism (i.e., water going into sweat and urine)
-shortness of breath   -cough
-sweating problems   -chest distention
-sputum   -allergies
-asthma

Kidneys

-dominates body fluid   -rules ears, hearing
-rules bones, including teeth

-vitality and moistness of head hair
-rules reproduction, growth and development
-stores essence which produces marrow: spinal cord,
  bone marrow, brain and manufactures blood and Essence

-sterility
-brittle bones
-stiffness of spine
-premature ejaculation
-premature grey hair
-joint pains, knee pains

-impotence
-urination
-low back ache
-receives Chi (air)

Spleen

-rules lips, eyelids
-opens to the mouth
-rules muscles, flesh and four limbs
-governs blood (keeps blood in the pathways)
-keeps internal organs in place
-transforms essence of food and fluids into Chi and
  Blood and, therefore, is the source of sufficient
  Blood and Chi in the body
-governs transformation and transportation, digestion,
  absorption and appetite

-sense of taste
-helps create blood

-abdominal distension or pain
-indigestion, gas and bloating
-uterine bleeding
-vomiting of blood, blood in stool, blood under skin,

-prolapse
-diarrhea
-anorexia

Liver

-rules tendons, nails
-rules menstrual flow
-regulates volume of circulation blood
-harmonizes emotions, even disposition
-rules smooth flow of Chi, smooth movement of bodily
  substances and regulation of body activities
  (maintains evenness and harmony of movement)

-opens to the eyes
-stores blood

-flank pain   -stagnation
-dizziness, numbness   -moving pains
-jaundice, bitter taste in mouth
-pain, distension or tightness in flanks
-swollen or painful breasts or genitals
-anger, depression, irritability, frustration

if invades spleen:

the above plus:

-abdominal pain   -nausea
-intestinal rumblings   -diarrhea
-belching

Pericardium

-protects heart   -attached to heart
-relationships (i.e., emotional counterparts to the heart)

YANG ORGANS

The Yang organs function to transform and dispose food and waste in the body.

Small Intestines

-Separates the pure from the impure
-receives and temporarily stores partially digested
 food from the stomach
-transfers residues with fluid to large intestines
-intestinal rumblings   -ulcers
-possibly bladder infections (fire of Heart shifted to Small
Intestines)   -unclarity

Large Intestines

-receives waste material from the Small Intestines
-absorbs fluids from the waste material

-excretes feces
-intestinal rumblings

-constipation
-diarrhea

Stomach

-spleen and stomach are source of health
-receives and decomposes food (sea of food and fluids)
-digestion and absorption
-vomiting
-indigestion

-it's Chi descends
-belching
-ulcers

Gallbladder

-rules decision making
-excretes bile into intestines to help digestion
-helps liver in promoting smooth flow of Chi

-stores bile

-jaundice

-spasms

Urinary Bladder

-stores and discharges urine
-urinary dysfunctions

Triple Warmer

Upper Warmer: Heart and Lungs
-transports Chi and Blood to nourish body
-like an all-pervading vapor or mist
Middle Warmer: Spleen, Stomach and Intestines
-digestion and absorption
-like a foam, or soaking things in water
Lower Warmer: Kidneys, Urinary Bladder and Liver
-controls water metabolism and storage and
excretion of urine
-like a swamp, and pathway for the flowing of water

EXTRAORDINARY ORGANS

Brain

The brain is the sea of marrow. It's primary
functions are:

-memorization   -thinking

These four organs are directly involved with the brain:

Kidneys: essence for the brain comes from the
kidneys
Heart: houses the mind and dominates thinking
Liver: rules smooth flow of vital functions
Spleen: rules concentration

Uterus

The uterus presides over menstruation and nourishes the fetus. These organs are involved:

Kidneys: includes essence, menstruation, conception and fetal growth
Liver: regulates volume of blood circulation
Spleen: produces blood, keeps blood in the vessels

14.DISEASE SYNDROMES

Patterns of disharmony involving particular Organs are primarily a synthesis of the Syndromes of Chi, Yang, Blood and Yin, the Pernicious Influences, and the signs and symptoms corresponding to the individual Organs. All of these manifest together in various combinations and form a variety of pattern sequences.

Here we list the patterns of disharmony commonly encountered in clinical practice as not all possible combinations of patterns are generally seen. Under each Organ is first listed the basic signs, symptoms and aspects ruled by that Organ. Next follows the specific pattern combinations most commonly seen for that Organ.

Because the Yin Organs provide the vital functions, they are the ones usually discussed. Patterns for the Yang Organs are generally disharmonies in those Organ's functions.

THE YIN ORGANS

Heart

Basic Signs:
- palpitations
- mind and mental activity
- blood, vessels and circulation
- opens to the tongue
- shen (spirit)
- insomnia

Patterns of disharmony:

Deficient heart chi

- weak and irregular pulse
- lethargy
- shortness of breath
- pale tongue
- palpitations
- muddled shen (spirit)

Note: This pattern often occurs with that of Deficient Lung Chi and/or Deficient Kidney yang.

Deficient Heart Yang

the same signs as Deficient Heart Chi, only more severe, plus,

-swollen, moist tongue
-other cold signs
-purplish lips
-possible clear urine
plus collapse of Heart Yang:
-profuse sweating
-extremely cold limbs or body

-chills
-pallor
-cold limbs

-minute pulse
-purple lips

Deficient Heart Blood

-palpitations
-insomnia
-disturbed sleep
-pale tongue
-pale, lusterless face
-hard to fall asleep

-forgetfulness
-excessive dreaming
-feeling of unease
-thin pulse
-dizziness
-lethargy

Note: this pattern often occurs with that of Deficient Spleen Chi

Deficient Heart Yin

the same signs as Deficient Heart Blood plus:

-reddish tongue
-warm palms and soles
-low grade fever
-agitated manner

-thin pulse
-malar flush
-night sweats
-easily awakened

Note: This pattern often occurs with that of Deficient Kidney Yin

Congealed Heart Blood

-palpitations
-purple face, lips and nails
-stabbing pain
-thready missed beat pulse
-dark purple tongue or purple spots on tongue
-if mucus is included, the tongue moss will be thick and greasy

-lassitude

-shortness of breath

Cold Mucus confusing the Heart Openings

-thick tongue moss
-abnormal behavior
talking to oneself
-sudden blackouts
-drooling

-slippery and slow pulse
-inward restrained manner
-staring at walls
-coma

Hot Mucus Confusing Heart Openings

-yellow thick tongue moss
-agitated manner
-incessant talking
-violent lashing out and other abnormal behaviors

-slippery, rapid pulse
-drooling

Hyperactivity of the Fire of the Heart

-hot and dark yellow urine
-insomnia with feverish sensation
-rapid pulse
-bitter taste in mouth
-swelling and pain of mouth and tongue

-ulceration
-flushed face
-red tongue

Lungs

Basic signs:

-cough
-chest distention
-protective chi (wei chi)
-skin and body hair

-shortness of breath
-sweating problems
-nose
-mucus in throat, vocal cords

Patterns of disharmony:

Cold in Lungs (external)

-chills
-head and body aches
-thin, white tongue moss
-stuffy, runny nose
-thin, watery sputum

-slight fever
-no perspiration
-floating tight pulse
-asthma or cough

Heat in Lungs (external)

-fever
-thirst
-slight chills
-constipation
-dry or bleeding nose

-perspiration
-dark urine
-fast pulse
-shortness of breath

-red, sore swollen throat and\or with dry yellow moss
-asthmatic breathing or full cough with yellow sticky yellow expectorant
-runny nose with thick yellow phlegm
-expectorate bloody foul   -smelling pus

Wind in Lungs (external)

-itchy throat and cough   -possible fever and chills

Plus cold:
-more chills   -nasal obstruction
-mucoid sputum
-thin white tongue coating-watery nasal discharge

Plus Heat:

-more fever,   -redness and swelling of throat
-yellow tongue coating,   -sore throat
-purulent nasal discharge and sputum

Deficient Lung Chi

-weak respiration
-lowered resistance to colds
-low voice and lack of desire to talk
-exhausted appearance and spirit

-weak cough
-daytime sweats

Deficient Lung Yin

-bloody sputum
-thin, rapid pulse
-red cheeks-malar flush
-night sweats
-afternoon fever
-reddish tongue with dry moss
-dry cough, unproductive or with sticky scanty sputum
-feverish sensation in palms and soles of feet

-emaciated appearance
-low voice

-dry mouth

Damp Phlegm in Lungs

-shortness of breath
-sputum expectorant
-full high pitched pitched coughing
-wheezing or asthma with copious phlegm
-chest and flank distention and soreness
-increased difficulty in breathing when lying down
-thick greasy or sticky tongue moss, white or yellow

-slippery pulse

Note: This pattern is often seen with that of Deficient Spleen or Kidney Chi

Spleen

Basic signs:
-digestion
-abdominal distention or pain
-muscles/flesh

-diarrhea
-anorexia
-prolapse

-blood out of the pathways
-mouth, lips, taste, eyelids

Patterns of disharmony:

Deficient Spleen chi

-poor appetite   -loose stools
-empty pulse   -edema
-lethargy, lassitude-pale tongue with thin white moss
-slight abdominal pain and distention, relieved by touching
-blood out of vessels (such as bloody nose, blood in urine, stool, etc.)

Plus sinking chi:
-prolapse   -hemorrhage
-urinary incontinence
-extreme chronic diarrhea

Deficient Spleen Yang

the above plus:
-swollen moist pale tongue
-slow frail pulse   -cold limbs
-difficult urination   -edema
-other cold signs   -leukorrhea
-watery stools with undigested food
-abdominal distention and pain responds well to heat

Dampness in spleen

-lack of appetite   -nausea
-no sensation of taste   -watery stool
-slippery pulse   -borborygmus
-general lassitude   -abdominal pain
-no thirst or desire to drink-watery skin eruption
-thick greasy tongue moss-heaviness in head or body
-feeling of fullness in chest, head or epigastric region

Damp Heat in Spleen

-above plus:
-heat signs   -bitter taste in mouth
-jaundice

Spleen Unable to govern Blood

-bleeding, in stool, nose, hemorrhaging, excessive menses, uterine, etc.
-if with excess, there'll be heat in the blood, too

Note: this is usually seen with Deficient Spleen Chi or Yang-

Turbid Mucus disturbing the Head

the above plus:
-severe dizziness   -very greasy tongue moss

Liver

Basic signs:

-smooth flow of chi and blood   -stagnation
-pain or distention in flanks   -vision
-bile: jaundice, bitter taste   -numbness
-low abdominal pain   -heavy menses
-nails, tendons   -dizziness
-swollen or painful breasts or genitals
-emotional swings, anger, irritability

Patterns of Liver disharmony:

Deficient Liver Blood

-pale lusterless face
-blurring of vision
-pale fingernails
-dizziness   -dryness of eyes
-flank pain   -thin pulse

-hazy vision or spots in visual field
-irregular or insufficient menses or amenorrhea with prolonged cycle
-tendons and muscles numb, weak or has spasmodic movement

Deficient Liver Yin

Above plus:
-muddled vision
-wiry rapid thin pulse
-afternoon fever
-hot palms and soles

-red cheeks
-reddish tongue
-depression
-nervous tension

Liver Fire Rising

-splitting headaches
-red face and eyes
-eye diseases
-red tongue, yellow coat
-wiry rapid pulse
-hematemisis
-dark scanty urine
-deafness or sudden ringing in ears
-emotional outbursts, frequent anger
-distending sensation in head
-bitter taste in mouth

-insomnia
-epitaxis
-dry mouth
-hypertension
-irritability
-dizziness

Arrogant Liver Yang

This is a combination of Excess Fire and Deficient Yin:

-throbbing headache
-reddish eyes, some pain
-anger or depression
-periodic hot flushes in head and face

-some dizziness
-rapid wiry pulse

Constrained Liver Chi

-wiry or tight pulse
-discomfort in chest
-blue-green, purplish or darkish tongue

-lump in throat
-belching, sighing

-depression, frustration, inappropriate anger
-distention or lumps in breast, groin or neck
-hypochondriac or low abdominal pain
-menstrual pain, irregular menses

Liver invades spleen

the above plus:
-nausea   -vomiting
-abdominal pain   -diarrhea
-no tiredness here   -sour belching

Liver Wind

-trembling   -difficulty in speech
-stiff neck or tetany
-pulsating headaches
-extreme dizziness   -tinnitus
-wiry rapid pulse   -spasms
-convulsions   -coma
-facial rigidity or twitching
-unconsciousness (apoplexy)
-deep red or purplish tongue

Cold in Liver

-deep slow and wiry pulse
-pain and distention in lower side and groin
-heat relieves pain
-swollen scrotum with bearing-down sensation
-pale moist tongue with white moss

Kidney

Basic signs:

-ears, hearing   -head hair
-premature grey hair   -reproduction

-joint pains, knee pains   -low back pain
-bones and marrow, tooth problems
-urinary problems
-growth and development   -head hair
-Essence: sterility, impotence, brittle bones,
-stiffness of spine, weak legs and knees

Patterns of disharmony:

Deficient Kidney Chi

-frequent urination   -enuresis
-incontinence of urine   -polyuria
-soreness and weakness of lower back and knees
-dribbling of urine after urination

Plus: possible infertility, shortness of breath, asthma, thready pulse

Deficient Kidney Yang

Signs of Deficient Kidney Chi plus:

-night urination   -cold limbs
-edema of lower limbs   -loose teeth
-general debilitation   -fear of cold
-spermatorrhea   -no shen (spirit)
-copious clear urine   -dribbling urine
-impotence, sterility
-subdued quiet manner
-minute, slow or frail pulse
-bright, white or darkish face
-cold and sore lower back and knees
-swollen pale tongue with scallops
-deafness or loss of hearing
-moist, thin white tongue moss

With Deficient Heart Yang: edema and Heart palpitations
With Deficient Spleen Yang: edema, chronic digestive problems
With Deficient Lung Chi: Chronic cough, shortness of breath or asthma

Deficient Kidney Yin

-thin, emaciated
-hot palms and soles
-weak sore back
-blurring of vision
-hot deep yellow urine
-thin rapid pulse
-premature ejaculation
-forgetfulness
-constipation
-reddish tongue with little moss
-ringing in ears or loss of hearing

-vertigo
-night sweats
-dry throat
-poor memory
-night sweating
-malar flush
-tinnitus
-dizziness
-little sperm

Deficient Kidney Essence

The regular Kidney signs plus:

-no hot or cold signs
-dry vaginal secretions
-nocturnal emission
-premature aging or senility
-infertility
-sexual dysfunction, impotence, sterility

-bad teeth
-brittle bones
-poor memory

Pericardium

Basic signs:

-protects heart

-relationships

Patterns of Pericardium disharmony:

-high fever
-possible derangement of the mind, coma

-delirium

THE YANG ORGANS

Small Intestines

Basic signs:

-digestion and absorption
-separating pure from impure
Patterns of Small Intestine disharmony:

Heat being transferred from the heart to the small intestine
-the same signs as in the pattern of Hyperactivity of the Fire of the Heart and usually includes blood in the urine.

Large intestines

Basic signs:

-absorbs fluids from waste material
-constipation   -diarrhea
-intestinal rumblings   -excretes feces

Patterns of Large Intestine disharmony:

-fever   -abdominal pain
-frequent bowel movements   -tenesmus
-loose dark stools with offensive smell
-burning sensation of the anus
-possible white and red mucus in stool

Stasis of the Large Intestine

-distension and fullness in the abdomen
-nausea   -constipation
-vomiting
-abdominal pain intensified upon pressure

Stagnation of Blood and Heat in the Large intestine
-severe or drilling fixed pain in the lower abdomen
-constipation or mild diarrhea
-possible fever and vomiting

Stomach

-digestion and absorption
-indigestion
-belching

-vomiting
-nausea

Patterns of Stomach disharmony:

-distension and pain in epigastric region
-sour regurgitation
-possible vomiting

-foul belching
-loss of appetite

Retention of Fluid in the Stomach due to Cold

-fullness and dull pain in the epigastric region aggravated by cold
-vomiting of watery fluid
-shortness of breath
-restlessness
-profuse sweating
-depletion of fluids

-heat stroke
-disturbed mind
-exhaustion

Gallbladder

Basic signs:

-stores bile
-rules decision making

-spasms
-jaundice

Patterns of Gallbladder disharmony:

Damp-Heat in the Gallbladder

-bright yellow sclera and skin
-possible: pain in costal and hypochondriac region or right upper abdomen with bitter taste in the mouth, vomiting of sour and bitter fluid

Urinary Bladder

Basic signs:

-stores and discharges urine
-urinary dysfunctions

Damp-Heat in the Urinary Bladder

-frequent and urgent urination
-burning pain upon urination
-scanty and difficult urination with possible reddish tinge or signs of blood
-possible blood clots or stones in urine

Disturbance in the Function of the Urinary Bladder

-dribbling urination   -weak stream
-intolerance to cold   -pale face
-retention of urine
-weakness of lumbar region and knee joints

Triple Warmer

Basic signs:

Upper Warmer: signs of the Heart and Lung
Middle Warmer: signs of the Spleen, Stomach and Intestines
Lower Warmer: signs of the Kidney, Urinary Bladder and Liver

Patterns of Triple Warmer disharmony:

Triple Warmer syndromes are involved in syndromes of the yin and yang organs relating to the upper, middle and lower warmers as listed above. Obstruction of the upper warmer, for example, refers to constrainment of lung chi; deficient chi of the middle warmer refers to weakness of the spleen and stomach; damp-heat in the lower warmer means damp-heat in the urinary bladder.

15. METHODS OF EXAMINATION

The examination methods in Oriental Medicine act as a bridge between theory and treatment. It is through these methods that one determines the patterns of disharmony which are manifesting. Four examination methods are used: 1) looking, 2) listening/smelling, 3) asking and 4) touching. Together, these methods show what to look for, the significance of what is seen and how to interpret the signs and symptoms. By gathering all possible information from these sources, one sees a pattern begin to emerge which then points the direction for treatment.

It is important, however, to observe how every sign or symptom fits into the whole picture and then treat the entire pattern presented. If just individual correspondences are followed, then a misrepresentation can occur. For instance, a floating pulse usually denotes the invasion of an External Pernicious Influence. However, if this pulse occurs without strength, then it signifies a Deficient Yin condition. This is because the Yin is not holding the Yang down, and so it rises and is Yang active. The lack of strength shows that it is from a Deficient Yin condition, though, rather than a true Excess of Yang. Therefore, in examination all the signs and symptoms must be taken together and seen how they fit into a total pattern before a treatment approach is decided upon.

1) Looking

Looking includes observing several aspects of the person such as the overall spirit, appearance, skin color, posture, tongue and excretions and secretions. In general, if the person is in fairly good spirits and is responsive, then the disease is mild. If the person is spiritless and indifferent, then the disease is serious. In terms of facial color, red denotes Heat; pallor signifies Cold or Deficiency of Blood; bright yellow suggests jaundice; and bluish purple is stagnation of Blood or severe pain.

An emaciated person often has Deficiency of Yin and hyperactivity of Fire; an obese person often has Deficiency of Chi and much Phlegm-Damp. An aggressive, outward and talkative person tends toward Yang whereas a passive, introverted and quiet person is usually Yin. Heavy, forceful and aggressive movement is usually an Excess condition; frail and weak movement is generally Deficiency.

The Tongue

The tongue is divided into the tongue material itself and the coating of the tongue, called moss or fur. These two are taken separately when examining the tongue. A normal tongue is pale red, somewhat moist, free in motion and with a thin layer of white coating. A pale tongue indicates Deficient Blood, Deficient Chi or Excess Cold, whereas a red tongue signifies Heat. A purple tongue, or tongue with purple spots indicates stagnation of Chi and Blood. It also indicates internal Cold due to Deficiency of Yang.

A flabby tongue is larger than normal, flabby and whitish in color, sometimes with teeth prints on the border. This indicates a Deficiency of both Chi and Yang and retention of Damp. A deep red flabby tongue indicates hyperactivity of Heart Fire. A cracked tongue has irregular streaks or cracks on the tongue (this does not include those from birth) and points to excessive Heat, loss of Kidney Essence and hyperactivity of Fire due to Yin Deficiency. A trembling tongue indicates Wind or Deficient Chi.

A thin coating on the tongue is normal, but when seen with a disease, it may be from a Deficiency, A very thick moss is usually a sign of Excess. Tongue fur that is streaked with moisture shows Dampness or possibly Deficient Yang. Dry Moss is a sign of Excess Yang or Fire, or of Deficient Fluids. Greasy moss is like a thick, oily film. It signifies Dampness, or Phlegm if it is extreme. Moss which seems to have been removed so that the tongue appears shiny, signifies Deficient Yin or Fluids.

White moss with an illness signifies Cold if there is excessive moisture in the tongue material. But white moss resembling cottage cheese signifies Heat in the stomach. A yellow moss denotes Heat. A black or gray moss is either extreme Heat or Cold, extreme Heat if the tongue material is red, extreme Cold if it is pale.

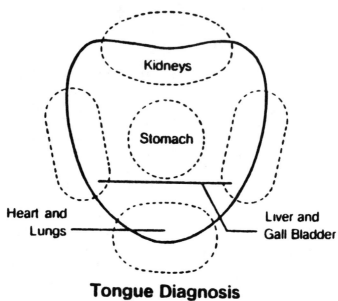

Tongue Diagnosis

2) <u>Listening and Smelling</u>

The next examination is listening to the person's breathing and mode of speech and cough, and smelling the body odors. In Deficient syndromes the breathing is shallow and soft; rough, heavy breathing occurs in Excess diseases. Speech and wheezing are differentiated as Excessive or Deficient in the same manner. A gurgling cough is Phlegm-Damp; a weak one is Deficiency; a violent sudden heavy cough is Excess; a dry, hacking cough is usually Dryness and Heat.

Offensive, foul or rancid smells from discharges or excretions usually indicate Heat syndromes of the Excess type, while Cold and Deficiency diseases may smell pungent or like rotten fish. Congestion of food may cause the person to have rotten, sour breath.

3) Asking

Asking the person pertinent questions is an important way to obtain information that is not readily available. Many, many questions may be asked, but only those that are the most essential to pattern perception are covered here. This information must, however, be combined with the other methods of examination to form an accurate overall pattern of disharmony.

a) Main Complaint

b) Health History - include the parent's

c) Chills and Fever - if these appear together then they indicate an External Pernicious Influence. If the chills are stronger, it is a Wind/Cold disease; if the fever is stronger it is a Wind/Hot condition. Alternating Chills and Fever is Half Exterior/Half Interior conditions. If the fever rises during the night the condition is serious. A Deficient Yin condition develops a low fever daily or a feeling of heat in the soles and palms in the afternoon or evening, which breaks late at night into a sweat.

d) Perspiration - Heavy sweating during the day indicates Deficient Chi; Heavy sweating at night signifies Deficient Yin. If there is not perspiration during an illness with fever and other External signs, then Cold has obstructed the pores. A lot of perspiration during an External condition signifies Heat. If the fever breaks after perspiration, the Pernicious Influence has been expelled.

e) Pain and Headaches - Pain manifesting in a particular part of the body indicates a disharmony in that area. Pain helped by heat is from Cold; if it is diminished by cold it is Heat. If it is relieved by touch or pressure it is from Deficiency; if it is aggravated by touch or pressure it is Excess. If it is sharp and stabbing, and usually fixed in location, it is congealed Blood. If it moves from place to place, it is Wind or Stagnant Chi. If it has a sensation of heaviness, it is Damp.

Severe headaches may be a sign of Excess, while slight, annoying headaches are usually signs of Deficiency. When the head feels under a lot of pressure, it is Dampness. Frontal headaches are associated with the stomach and large intestine; behind the hairline with the small intestine and urinary bladder; at the vertex with the liver; at the sides of the head with the gallbladder.

f) Urine and Stool - Excessive urination is due to Deficient kidney Yang; clear urine is a Cold pattern while dark yellow or reddish urine indicates Heat. Scanty urination usually is due to an Excess, such as Damp-Heat in the Bladder.

Infrequent, hard or dry stools indicate Heat, but may also denote Deficient Fluids or Deficient Chi. Watery or unformed and frequent stools are usually Deficient Chi, Deficient Yang, or Dampness. Massive and sudden diarrhea is a condition of Excess. Long-term diarrhea results from Deficient Spleen.

g) Diet, Appetite and Thirst - Not being thirsty or desiring warm drinks, indicates Cold. A lot of thirst, especially for cool drinks, indicates Heat. Lack of thirst or thirst with no desire to drink points to Dampness. A good appetite shows the disease is not too serious. Lack of appetite with a bloated feeling after eating is either a weak Spleen or Damp Heat. Stomach Heat can cause constant hunger.

A bitter taste in the mouth suggests Heat, usually of the liver or gall bladder. A sweet pasty taste indicates Damp Heat in the spleen. Foul taste usually means stomach or liver Heat. Inability to taste is generally due to Deficient spleen Chi.

Usually here it is a good idea to find out what kinds of foods the person has been and is now eating. This helps point to the potential pattern that has developed in the body. Often if a person does not change the diet, then it takes much longer for the disharmony to be righted.

h)   Sleep - insomnia or restless sleep is generally Deficient Heart Blood or Yin. Excessive sleepiness may be due to Deficient Yang, Deficient Chi or Dampness.

i) Menses and Leukorrhea - Early periods suggest Heat, while late ones indicate Deficient Blood or Cold causing Stagnation. Irregular menstruation is often a sign of irregular Liver Chi. Excessive menses may be Heat in the Blood or Deficient Chi. Insufficient flow or lack of menses may mean Deficient Blood, Cold obstructing the Blood or Congealed Blood. Very dark blood indicates Heat, while pale and thin blood point to Deficiency. Purplish blood, especially if clotted, may indicated Congealed Blood. Pain before the period is from Excess, while after the period has started it is from Deficiency.
Copious, clear or white and thin discharges are generally from Deficiency and Dampness. Thick and yellow discharges, usually with itching of the vagina, are often from Damp-Heat.

j)   Emotional Tendencies - There are seven emotions recognized in Chinese medicine. They are joy (heart), anger (liver), sadness and grief (lung), pensiveness (spleen), and fear and fright (kidney). Emotional excess or insufficiency affects the Fundamental Substances and the Organs. Excessive anger damages the liver, resulting in dizziness, chest congestion, red eyes and a bitter taste in the mouth. Likewise, an imbalanced organ can cause a particular emotion to be prominent, such as a disharmonious lung causing a person to be overly sad or grieving.

4) Touching

In the palpation part of the examination the pulse is felt and particular points on the body may be pressed, such as the Alarm (Mu) Points and Associated Effect (Shu) Points. One can also feel for a sensation of hot, cold, or dryness on the skin, abnormal masses, or if pain is diminished or aggravated by pressure.

The Pulse

Taking the pulse is a subtle art and there are as many as 28 different pulses. Yet, it is possible to learn six major differentiations of the pulse that can give a general but useful picture. Take at least 5 to 10 pulses to gain a general understanding of each type of pulse. The pulses are taken at the radial artery near the wrist. Place your middle finger parallel to the lower knob on the posterior of the radius. The index finger will then automatically fall next to the wrist, and the ring finger will fall next to the middle finger, the farthest away from the wrist.

There are three positions felt on each hand, with the index finger touching the first (1) position, the middle finger touching the second (2) position and the ring finger touching the third (3). Organs are generally assigned to each of the pulse positions of the left and right hands, with the Yin organs felt at the deep position and the Yang organs felt at the superficial position. See the accompanying picture for details.

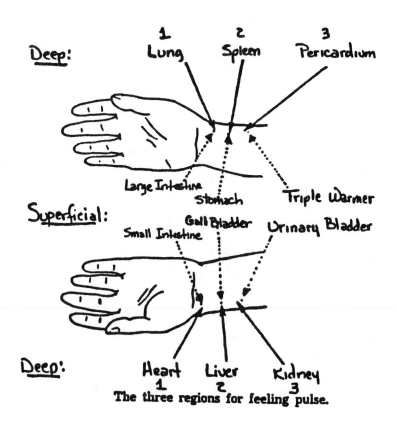

The three regions for feeling pulse.

1)   Depth: if the pulse is floating then this usually indicates an External Pernicious Influence. If it is floating and without strength, however, then this indicates Deficient Yin. A deep or submerged pulse indicates internal disharmonies and is classified as Yin.

2)   Speed: A slow pulse is one that has fewer than four beats per complete breath (this includes a normal inhalation and exhalation for the person whose pulse you are taking). It usually occurs in Cold syndromes. A rapid pulse is quick, with more than 5 beats per breath and often occurs in Heat syndromes.

3)   Strength: a Deficient pulse is weak, forceless and disappears on heavy pressure. It often occurs in syndromes of the Deficient type. A thin pulse which feels like a fine thread is Deficient Blood. An empty pulse is big but without strength. It feels weak and soft like a balloon partially filled with water. It is usually superficial and slower than normal. It signifies Deficient Chi and Blood. The Deficient pulse is classified as Yin.

An Excess pulse is forceful and is felt even on deep pressure. It often occurs in syndromes of the Excess type. The big pulse is broad in diameter and very distinct, whereas the full pulse is big and strong, pounding hard against the fingers at all three depths. The excess pulse is classified as Yang.

From these six pulses one can determine if the pattern is Internal or External, Deficient or Excess, Hot or Cold, and Yin or Yang.

PART III - THERAPIES

Treating the patterns of Organ disharmony can be simple to complicated depending on the person and how the disharmony manifests. In general, if there is an excess, then eliminate; a Deficiency, then tonify; too much damp, then dry; if dry, then moisten; if cold, then add warmth; if hot, then cool; if windy, then pacify; if stuck, then move it; and if moving improperly, then regulate it. This is a highly simplified way of thinking about treating disharmonies, but gives the beginning basic approach.

16. THE THREE HUMOURS

a). BLOOD:
Herbal categories: tonify and move blood, nutritives, tonics, emmenagogues, alteratives, demulcents.
Formulas and foods: tonics and nutritives: number 6, 7 (Women's formula), 24 (Yin), Szu Wu Tang, 29 (Precious herbs), Gui Pi Tang, bone marrow soup, Black beans, dark grapes.
Moving blood and emmenagogues: 6, 7 (women's formulas), Szu Wu Tang, wine, ginger, wild ginger, pennyroyal, spices such as oregano, marjoram, thyme, etc.
Cool heated blood and alteratives: Formulas numbers 14, 15 (blood purifiers), 12 (liver), also mung beans, fresh green vegetables, fruit.

b). Fluid:
Herbal categories: Tonify Yin, nutritives, demulcents, emollients, tonics, vulneraries, diuretics, expectorants, cholagogues.
Formulas and foods: formulas numbers 24 (Yin), marshmallow root, slippery elm bark, comfrey root, oysters, barley, oats, wheat gluten, okra.
Diuretics: formula number 2 (diuretic), parsley leaves and root, barley, azuki red beans, mushrooms.

Expectorants: Old Indian syrup, locquat leaves and fruit, pears, garlic, onions, yerba santa, fritillary bulbs.
Cholagogues: Formula number 12 (liver), dandelion root, endive, chicory, barberry root and oregon grape root.

c). Chi:
  Herbal categories: Chi tonic, regulate Chi, carminatives.
  Formulas and foods: formulas numbers 22 (ginseng complex), Chyavanprash, Eight Precious herbs, ginseng, astragalus, codonopsis, atractylodes, oats, dates, raw brown sugar, red meat, cooked whole grains.
  Regulate Chi and Carminatives: formula number 20 (Hingashtak), Liver Chi regulating formula, anise seed, fennel seed, dill seed, radish, parsley.

17. SIX STAGES OF DISEASE

1. Greater Yang (Tai Yang):
  Herbal categories: diaphoretics, warming stimulants.
  Formulas and foods: Formula number 16 (composition formula), elder flower and mint tea, fresh ginger tea, cayenne pepper, garlic tea, raw brown sugar tea, basil tea, oregano tea.

2. Lesser Yang (Hsiao Yang):
  Herbal categories: harmonizing therapies can combine opposite principles from many categories in the same formula such as herbs and foods that both eliminate and build, warm and cool, relax and stimulate, etc..
  Formulas and Foods: Minor Bupleurum Tea (This versatile traditional formula is one of the most frequently indicated and useful, it treats hypoglycemia, and various prolonged inflammatory symptoms including asthma, bronchitis and flu), combinations of Formulas numbers 12 and number 8 (antistress formula) or number 22 (ginseng complex formula); combinations of both numbers 24 (Yin) and number 25 (Yang) formulas; combinations of number 6 or number 7 (Women's Formulas) and number 12 (liver) and/or number 8 (Stress).

83

3. Sunlight Yang (Yang Ming):
    Herbal Categories: Purgatives.
    Formulas and foods: number 19 (Triphala), cascara bark, rhubarb root, senna leaves, stewed dates, olive oil, fruits and fruits juices.

4. Greater Yin (Tai Yin):
    Herbal Categories: internal warming and tonics.
    Formulas and foods: Numbers 31 (warmth), number 18 (Trikatu), number 22 (ginseng complex), cayenne pepper, garlic, ginger.

5. Lesser Yin (Hsiao Yin):
    Herbal Categories: Similar to the above.

6. Absolute Yin (Chueh Yin):
    Herbal categories: Similar to the two previous.

18. EIGHT METHODS OF HERBAL TREATMENT

1. Sweating:
    Herbal Categories: Surface relieving, cooling or warming diaphoretics.
    Formulas: Number 16 (composition formula) take two or more tablets with warm water immediately at the first sign of upper respiratory infection, cold, and flu. For sore throats Herbal Uprising should be made into a warm infusion and taken freely, even gargling to clear the throat.

    Tea: Elder flowers, Mint, Yarrow --1/3 ounce of each steeped in a pint of water, take before a hot bath and/or going to bed to sweat. About 20 or 30 minutes after sweating therapy replenish a weakened patient's strength by feeding a bowl of thin rice congee (made with 7 cups or more of water to one cup of rice and cooked slowly in a double boiler or slow cooker for 6 to 8 hours) or some other appropriate easily digested whole grain cereal. This can be mildly sweetened with honey or barley malt syrup if desired. Especially good for children is a tea of lemon balm (melissa officinalis).
    One should be careful to not sweat to extreme exhaustion. It is a good idea to supplement the energy by giving a warm rice porridge an hour or so after sweating.

2. Vomiting:

Herbal categories: Nauseants.

Herbal treatments: Lobelia emetic, Syrup of Ipecac, drinking two or three cups of strong licorice tea or warm salt water can be used to induce vomiting. While vomiting therapy is good for food poisoning, it should not be used for poisoning caused by the ingestion of caustic chemicals. For this type of poisoning one should use demulcent herbs such as marshmallow root or slippery elm bark or boiled warm milk. In any case, try to obtain qualified medical help.

3. Purging:

Herbal category: purgatives and laxatives.

Herbal treatments: Formula number 19 (Triphala), one of the best and safest bowel regulators. For occasional use take 3 to 4 tablets in the evening with warm water. For blood purification and ongoing bowel regulation take two or more tablets three times daily. To prevent any dryness of the bowels be sure to drink at least 8 ounces of warm water with Triphala.

For stronger purges, extracts of cascara sagrada, senna or rhubarb can be given with ginger tea to prevent griping. Lubricating laxatives are used for intestinal dryness. For this use psyllium seeds and/or husks, flax seed or a combination of both with chia seeds as a supplementing tonic (I call this Three Seeds Bowel Tonic). Take a tablespoon of each steeped either in licorice tea or black cherry juice before going to bed in the evening.

For children, steep a tablespoon of manuka raisins (the large ones) in a cup of Licorice tea and give before going to bed in the evening. For women experiencing cramping and blood clots in the pelvic region a combination of Formulas number 19 (Triphala) and number 6 (Women's Formula) should be taken three times a day with ginger and chamomile tea.

Contraindications for purgative therapies is if the condition is a true Greater Yang surface condition as purging internally can further weaken one's defenses to fight off the external pathogen.

4. Harmonizing:
    Herbal category: combination therapies.
    Formulas and foods: Minor Bupleurum Combination, various combinations of formulas number 12 (liver) and number 8 (Stress); number 12 (liver) and number 6 or number 7 (Women's Formula), number 12 (liver) and 22 (Ginseng complex).
    Harmonizing therapy is not appropriate for individuals with an external or internal disease.

5. Warming:
    Herbal categories: Warming stimulants.
    Formulas and foods: number 18 (Trikatu), number 31 (warmth), number 16 (Composition Formula), number 20 (HingaShtak), number 23 (Flexibility) cayenne and black peppers, horseradish, angelica root, lamb.
    Warming therapy is contraindicated for individuals with excess heat, fast pulse, flushing of the complexion and feelings of burning or heat. It should be used very carefully for individuals with wasting heat diseases.

6. Removing:
    Herbal categories: heat clearing, alteratives, cholagogues.
    Formulas and foods: numbers 14 and 15 (blood purifiers), 12 (skin clearing), 4 (prostate), echinacea, 11 (Diet Complex), 19 (Triphala), 12 (liver), mung beans, green vegetables, juices and fruits.

7. Supplementing:
    Herbal categories: tonics.
    Formulas and foods: numbers 22 (Ginseng Complex), 21 (Chyavanprash), 6 (Women's Formula), 30 (Wu Zi Wan), 29 (precious Herbs), Ginseng and Antler combination, 32 (Buzhong Elixir), Szu Wu Tang, Si Junza Tang, 24 (Yin) And 25 (Yang), 28 (Jade Screen), meat, root vegetables, cooked whole grains.
    Contraindications are for those with excess and stagnant conditions, with acute, feverish diseases, constipation and inflammatory diseases.

8. Reducing:
   Herbal categories: alteratives, diuretics, purgatives, diaphoretics, expectorants.
   Formulas and foods: numbers 11 (Diet Program), 19 (Triphala), 3 (stone removing), 2 (Diuretic), 1 (Decongestant). Contraindications for reducing therapies is for those with weakness of Chi, abdominal distension, low grade fever, thirst, loss of appetite, diarrhea, weak digestion, individuals with severe loss of blood.

19. HERBAL SYNDROMES TREATMENTS

Treating the patterns of Organ disharmony is a process of deduction based upon the various criteria of differential diagnosis previously outlined. Thus, if there is excess, then eliminate with alteratives, cholagogues or purgatives; for deficiency, tonify selecting yang, yin, chi or blood tonics; if dry, moisten with demulcents, emollients and yin or blood tonics; if cool, then warm with stimulants; if hot, then cool with diaphoretics, alteratives, purgatives or cholagogues; if wind or tension manifests, then pacify with nervines and antispasmodics; if stuck or congested, then move with emmenagogues or stimulants; if moving is not smooth or regular, then regulate with carminatives.

Acute diseases generally manifest or are treated more simply using primarily one approach as indicated. Chronic diseases are more complex and must be treated more 'holistically', addressing several aspects of the problem simultaneously with appropriate emphases for each. Of course, one cannot ignore the importance of the subtler aspects of intuition in arriving at a proper diagnosis but the point to remember is that diagnosis will always be the key to successful treatment.

What is generally not understood is that this fundamental approach to healing is predicated upon the use of relatively mild food-like herbs. Since they have relatively few or no side effects, it is only with herbs that one can undergo such a comprehensive approach to 'holistic' treatment as drugs are too strong and carry high risks of dangerous side effects. The reason such chronic degenerative diseases as heart disease, cancer, arthritis are difficult to cure with Western drugs is that these diseases usually involve the degeneration and breakdown of

87

several systems simultaneously and chemical drugs tend to be too specific.

Following are some suggested formulas and treatment approaches for the patterns of Organ disharmony previously described.

PERNICIOUS INFLUENCES

Wind:

Herbal Categories:
External: Surface Relieving, Spicy Warm or Cold
Internal: Extinguish Draft, Relieve Spasm
Wind-Damp: Eliminate Draft Wet
Formulas: 8 (StressFree), 9 (HeadAid formula), 6 (Calm Child)
Herbs and Foods: Camomile, Skullcap herb, Calcium, Magnesium

Cold:

Herbal Categories:
External: Surface Relieving, Spicy Warm
Internal: Warm Interior, Eliminate Cold, Tonify Yang
Formulas: 25 (TaiChi Ginseng Complex), 22 (Royal Tonic or Chyavanprash), 17 (Composition formula or Herbal Uprising), 19 (Trikatu), 37 (Herbal Warmth)
Herbs and Foods: Ginger, Cinnamon, Cloves, Cayenne; Red Meat, Lamb

Heat:

Herbal Categories:
External: Surface Relieving Spicy Cool
Internal: all five Clear Heat categories, Purge Attack
Formulas: Echinacea, numbers 21 (Triphala), 14, 15 (blood purifiers), 4 (Witasu prostate formula), 12 (HepatoPure for the liver)
Herbs and Foods: Echinacea, Chaparral, Violet leaves, Burdock Root, Red Clover, Dandelion; Mung beans, Green vegetables, Fruit and Juices, Endive, Lettuce

Damp:

Herbal Categories:
External: Clear and Dissolve Cold or
Heated Phlegm, Relieve Cough and Asthma
Internal: above plus Promote Water Flow, Permeate
Wet, Fragrant-Dissolve Wet, Purge Diuretics
Cold Damp: add Warm Interior
Eliminate Cold, Tonify Yang
Damp Heat: add Clear Heat Dry Wet
Formulas: Numbers 13 (HerbaDerm), 2 (Diurite), 25
(TaiChi Ginseng Complex), 3 (Stone Free),19 (Trikatu),
1 (Breeze Free), 21 (Triphala), 17 (Herbal Uprising),
20 (HingaShtak), 12 (HepatoPure), 28 (Yang Tonic)
Herbs and Foods: Cleavers, Couchgrass, Parsley,
Juniper berries, Yerba santa, Locquat Leaves; Aduki
Beans

Dryness:

Herbal Categories: Tonify Yin, Purge-Lubricate
Formulas: Number 6 (Women's Treasure), 24 (Yin
Tonic) 14 (River of Life)
Other Formulas: 35 (Eight Precious Herbs)
Herbs and Foods: Gelatin, Marshmallow Root,
Comfrey Root, Licorice Root, Slippery Elm Bark; Oats,
Barley, Seaweed, Okra

Summer Heat:

Herbal Category: Clear Heat Relieve Summer Heat
Formulas: number 14 (River of Life), Echinacea, 8
(Stress Free)
Herbs and Foods: Mung Beans, Melon, Cucumber

Phlegm:

Herbal Categories: Clear and Dissolve Heated or Cool
Phlegm, Relieve Cough and Asthma
Formulas: Number 1 (Breeze Free), 25 (Tai Chi), 19
(Trikatu), 20 (HingaShtak)
Herbs and Foods: Cinnamon, Locquat Leaves, Mullein
Leaf, Elecampane Root; Honey, Pear

DIFFERENTIATION OF SYNDROMES

Deficient Chi:
    Herbal Category: Tonify Chi
    Formulas: 25 (Tai Chi Ginseng Complex)
    Other Formulas: 36 (Wu Zi Wan), 31 (Jade Screen)
    Herbs and Foods: Ginseng; Meat, Carrots, Dates,
    Raw Sugar, Garlic and/or Onions sauteed in Ghee
    (clarified butter)

Deficient Yang:
    Herbal Categories: Tonify Yang, Warm Interior,
    Eliminate Cold
    Formulas: 19 (Trikatu), 18 (Vital Balance), 25 (Tai Chi),
    28 (Yang Tonic)
    Other Formulas: 36 (Wu Zi Wan)
    Herbs and Foods: Spices such as whole Cayenne
    Peppers, Ginger, Cumin Seeds, Turmeric Root and
    Coriander, together sauteed in Ghee; Mochi, Rice, Red
    Meat, Lamb

Stagnant Chi:
    Herbal Categories: Regulate Chi, Remove Congestion,
    Purge Attack
    Formulas: 20 (HingaShtak), 17 (Herbal Uprising)
    19 (Trikatu), 37 (Herbal Warmth), 21 (Triphala)
    Herbs and Foods: Ginger, Cinnamon, Calamus root,
    Coriander seed, Asafoetida, Cardamom, spices in
    general

Deficient Blood:
    Herbal Category: Tonify Blood
    Formulas: 6 (Women's Treasure), 6 (Women's Comfort)
    10, (Life Pulse), 27 (Yin Tonic)
    Other Formulas: number 35 (Eight Precious Herbs)
    Herbs and Foods: Burdock Root (Macrobiotic "Tekka"),
    Gelatin, Angelica, beets, Liver, Grapes and Raisins,
    Cooking in Iron pots, Spinach.

Deficient Yin:
   Herbal Categories: Tonify Yin, Clear Heat Cool Blood
   Formulas: 6 (Women's Treasure), 27 (Yin Tonic)
   Other Formulas: 35 (Eight Precious Herbs)
   Herbs and Foods: Comfrey Root, Irish Moss,
   Marshmallow Root, Blue and Black berries, Seaweed
   Soup, Milk, Oysters and Shellfish, Lean Pork.

Congealed Blood:
   Herbal Category: Vitalize Blood
   Formulas: 10 (Life Pulse), 6 (Women's Treasure), and
   7 Women's Comfort)
   Other Formulas: 35 (Eight Precious Herbs) 26
   (Flexibility)
   Herbs and Foods: Turmeric, Cayenne, Cinnamon,
   Ginger, Prickly Ash Bark, Saffron, Calendula, Mugwort
   Herb

Hot Blood:
   Herbal Categories: Clear Heat Cool Blood, Regulate
   Blood (Hemostatics)
   Formulas: 14 (River of Life), Echinacea, 21 (Triphala),
   15 (Complete Pau D' Arco)
   Herbs and Foods: Aloe Vera, Shepherd's Purse,
   Pumpkin, Wheat, Tofu, Eggplant, Spinach, Mung Beans

Deficiency of Essence:
   Herbal Category: Tonify Yin
   Formulas: 27 (Yin Tonic) 28 (Yang Tonic)
   Other Formulas: 36 (Wu Zi Wan)
   Herbs and Foods: Ginseng; Bone Marrow Soup, Oxtail
   Soup

Deficient Chi and Blood:
   Herbal Categories: Tonify Chi and Tonify Blood
   Formulas: Use combinations of 25 (Tai Chi), 6
   (Women's Treasure), 10 (Life Pulse), 7 (Women's
   Comfort), 27 (Yin Tonic)
   Other Formulas: Use combinations of: 36 (Wu Zi Wan),

31 (Jade Screen), 35 (Eight Precious Herbs)
Herbs and Foods: Use combinations of Ginseng, Turmeric, Burdock Root, Carrots, Dates, Raw Sugar, Beets, Dang Quai

Deficient Yin and Yang:
Herbal Categories: Tonify Yin and Tonify Yang, Warm Interior Eliminate Cold
Formulas: Use combinations of 6 (Women's Treasure), 19 (Trikatu), 25 (Tai Chi Ginseng Complex), 18 (Vital Balance)
Other Formulas: Use combinations of: 35 (Eight Precious Herbs), 36 (Wu Zi Wan)
Herbs and Foods: Use combinations of Comfrey Root, Irish Moss, Seaweed Soup, Mochi, Rice, Red Meat, Lamb, Milk, Black and Blue Berries

Excess Yin:
Herbal Categories: Promote Water Flow, Permeate Wet, Purge, Diuretics, Fragrant Dissolve Wet
Formulas: 2 (Diurite), 3 (Stone Free), 19 (Trikatu), 17 (Herbal Uprising), 21 (Triphala), 1 (Breeze Free), 13 (HerbaDerm), 25 (TaiChi Ginseng Complex), 20 (HingaShtak), 12 (HepatoPure)
Herbs and Foods: Cinnamon, Ginger, Parsley, Celery, Asparagus, Radish, Black and Small Red Bean

Excess Yang:
Herbal Categories: Clear Heat
Formulas: 12 (HepatoPure), 14 (River of Life), 15 (Complete Pau D'Arco), 13 (HerbaDerm), 19 (Triphala), Echinacea
Herbs and Foods: Skullcap, Rhubarb stalks and root used as a laxative; Green Vegetables, Squash, Raw Fruits, Juices

DIFFERENTIATION OF ORGANS

Heart:
> Formulas: 10 (Life Pulse), 14 (River of Life), 17 (Herbal Uprising), 12 (HepatoPure)
> Other Formulas: 35 (Eight Precious Herbs)

Lungs:
> Formulas: 1 (Breeze Free), 19 (Trikatu), 25 (Tai Chi Ginseng Complex)
> other: 31 (Jade Screen)

Kidneys:
> Formulas: 1 (Diurite), 3 (Stone Free), 4 (Witasu), 13 (HerbaDerm), 27 (Yin Tonic), 28 (Yang Tonic)
> Other Formulas: 36 (Wu Zi Wan)

Spleen:
> Formulas: 25 (Tai Chi Ginseng Complex),
> 20 (HingaShtak),
> 19 (Trikatu), 6 (Women's Treasure), 31 (Jade Screen),
> 35 (Eight Precious Herbs)

Liver:
> Formulas: 12 (HepatoPure), 8 (Stress Free),
> 5 (Calm Child), 13 (HerbaDerm), 18 (Vital Balance),
> 6 (Women's Treasure),
> 7 (Women's Comfort), 21 (Triphala), 14 (River of Life),
> 9 (HeadAid)
> Other Formulas: Minor Bupleurum

SYNDROMES OF DISEASE

<u>Heart</u>

Deficient Heart Blood and Yin:
  <u>Herbal Categories</u>: Tonify Blood and Tonify Yin
  <u>Formulas</u>: 10 (Life Pulse), 6 (Women's Treasure), 27
  (Yin Tonic)
  Other Formulas: 35 (Eight Precious Herbs)
  <u>Herbs and Foods</u>: Seaweed Soup, Pork, Bone Marrow
Soup,
  Wheat
Deficient Heart Chi and Yang:
  <u>Herbal Categories</u>: Tonify Chi and Tonify Yang
  <u>Formulas</u>: 25 (Tai Chi Ginseng Complex)
  Other Formulas: 35 (Eight Precious Herbs)
  <u>Herbs and Foods</u>: Ginger, Garlic;
  Red Meat Soup

Congealed Heart Blood:
  <u>Herbal Category</u>: Vitalize Blood
  <u>Formulas</u>: 10 (Life Pulse)
  Other: 35 (Eight Precious Herbs)
  <u>Herbs and Foods</u>: Wild Ginger, Tansy,
  Motherwort Herb, Pennyroyal, Garlic

Cold Mucus Confusing the Heart Openings:
  <u>Herbal Categories</u>: Clear and Dissolve Cold Phlegm,
  Fragrant Open Orifices
  <u>Formulas</u>: 10 (Life Pulse), 19 (Trikatu), 21
  (Triphala)
  Other Formulas: 35 (Eight Precious Herbs)
  <u>Herbs and Foods</u>: Cayenne, Cinnamon,
  Calamus, Garlic, Ginger

  Hot Mucus Confusing the Heart Openings:
  <u>Herbal Categories</u>: Clear and Dissolve
  Heated Phlegm, Fragrant Open Orifices
  <u>Formulas</u>: 14 (River of Life), 21 (Triphala)
  <u>Herbs and Foods</u>: Heartsease, Violet

Leaf, Hawthorne

Hyperactivity of the Fire of the Heart:
Herbal Category: Clear Heat Purge Fire
Formulas: 14 (River of Life), 21 (Triphala)
Herbs and Foods: Violet, Hawthorne Fruit
and Leaf, Pansy Leaf

Lungs

Cold in Lungs (external):
Herbal Category: Surface Relieving Spicy Warm
Formulas: 17 (Herbal uprising), 1 (Breeze Free), 19
(Trikatu)
Other Formulas: Pueraria Combination
Herbs and Foods: Fresh Ginger, Angelica, Elecampane,
Garlic, Cinnamon, Cardamom, Onions

Cold in Lungs (internal):
Herbal Categories: Warm Interior Eliminate Cold,
Clear and Dissolve Cold Phlegm
Formulas: 19 (Trikatu), 25 (ginseng complex)
Other Formulas: 37 (Jade Screen)
Herbs and Foods: Dry Ginger, Garlic, Cinnamon,
Walnuts

Heat in Lungs (external):
Herbal Category: Surface Relieving Spicy Cool
Formulas: 1 (Breeze Free), 5 (Calm Child)
Other Formulas: Pueraria Combination
Herbs and Foods: Comfrey Leaf, Mullein; Lemon,
Oats, Barley

Wind in Lungs (external):
Herbal Categories: Surface Relieving Spicy Warm or
Cool, Extinguish Draft Relieve Spasm
Formulas: 17 (Herbal uprising), 8 (Stress Free),
5. (Calm Child)
Other Formulas: Pueraria Combination,
37 (Jade Screen)
Herbs and Foods: Kuzu Root Sauce, Oats, Barley,

Garlic, Green Onions.

Deficient Lung Chi:
> Herbal Category: Tonify Chi
> Formulas: 25 (Tai Chi Ginseng Complex)
> Other Formulas: 37 (Jade Screen)
> Herbs and Foods: Ginseng, Astragalus, Ginger;
> Meat Soup, Walnuts.

Deficient Lung Yin:
> Herbal Category: Tonify Yin
> Formulas: 27 (Yin Tonic)
> Herbs and Foods: Comfrey Root, Aralia, American
> Ginseng; Oats, Barley, Seaweed

Dampness in Lungs:
> Herbal Categories: Clear and Dissolve Cold or Heated
> Phlegm, Relieve Cough and Asthma, Remove
> Congestion
> Formulas: 19 (Trikatu), 1 (Breeze Free), 2 (Diurite)
> Other Formulas: 31 (Jade Screen),
> Pueraria Combination
> Herbs and Foods: Kuzu Root Sauce, Honey, Pumpkin,
> Radish, Garlic

Spleen

Deficient Spleen Chi and Yang:
> Herbal Categories: Tonify Chi, Tonify Yang, Warm
> Interior Eliminate Cold
> Formulas: 25 (Tai Chi Ginseng Complex), 20
> (HingaShtak)
> Other Formulas: 31 (Jade Screen)
> Herbs and Foods: Panax Ginseng, Aralia; Rice, Millet,
> Meat Soup, Ginger

Spleen Unable to Govern Blood:
> Herbal Categories: Regulate Chi, Regulate Blood
> (Hemostatics), Tonify Chi
> Formulas: 10 (Life Pulse)

96

Other Formulas: Dang Quai Gin,
Dang Quai and Gelatin
Herbs and Foods: Gelatin, Raspberry, Turmeric, Squaw
Vine

Dampness in Spleen:
Herbal Categories: Promote Water Flow Permeate Wet,
Fragrant Dissolve Wet, Purge Diuretic, Remove
Congestion
Formulas: 25 (Tai Chi Ginseng Complex), 20
(HingaShtak),
21 (Triphala), 2 (Diurite), 3 (Stone Free)
Other Formulas: 31 (Jade Screen)
Herbs and Foods: Elecampane, Parsley Root, Juniper
berries, Cubeb Berries, Parsley, Asparagus, Carrots,
Aduki Beans

Damp Heat in Spleen:
Herbal Categories: Promote Water Flow Permeate Wet,
Purge Diuretic, Clear Heat Dry Wet
Formulas: 13 (HerbaDerm), 4 (Witasu), 12
(HepatoPure)
Herbs and Foods: Oregon Grape, Dandelion Root,
Barberry, Golden Seal, Poke Root, Dandelion Root,
Cleavers; Mung and Black Beans

Turbid Mucus Disturbing the Head:
Herbal Categories: Remove Congestion, Extinguish
Draft
Relieve Spasms, Fragrant Dissolve Wet
Formulas: 2 (Diurite) 25 (Tai Chi), 8 (Stress Free),
19 (Trikatu), 9 (HeadAid)
Herbs and Foods: Ginger Tea, Calamus

Liver

Constrained Liver Chi:
Herbal Categories: Regulate Chi, Extinguish Draft
Relieve Spasms
Formulas: 12 (HepatoPure) and 8 (Stress Free)
Other Formulas: Minor Bupleurum
Herbs and Foods: Fennel Seed, Citrus Peel, Cyperus,

Green Vegetables

Deficient Liver Blood and Yin:
> Herbal Categories: Tonify Blood, Tonify Yin
> Formulas: 6 (Women's Treasure), 27 (Yin Tonic)
> Other Formulas: 35 (Eight Precious Herbs)
> Herbs and Foods: Comfrey Root; Seaweed, Blueberries

Liver Fire Rising:
> Herbal Categories: Use combinations of Regulate Chi,
> Extinguish Draft Relieve Spasms, Clear Heat Purge Fire
> Formulas: 14 (River of Life), 15 (Complete Pau D'
> Arco), 21 (Triphala), 12 (HepatoPure),
> 8 (Stress Free), 5 (Calm Child)
> Herbs and Foods: Self Heal, Red Clover, Chamomile,
> Oregon Grape; Green Vegetables

Arrogant Liver Yang:
> Herbal Categories: Use combinations of Regulate Chi,
> Extinguish Draft, Relieve Spasms, Clear Heat Cool
> Blood, Tonify Yin
> Formulas: 27 (Yin Tonic), 12 (HepatoPure), 8 (Stress
> Free), 5 (Calm Child), 15 (Complete Pau D'Arco),
> 21 (Triphala)
> Other Formulas: 29 (precious herbs)
> Herbs and Foods: Dandelion Root, Oregon Grape,
> Steamed Green Vegetables

Liver Wind:
> Herbal Categories: Extinguish Draft Relieve Spasms,
> Regulate Chi, Eliminate Draft Wet
> Formulas: 8 (Stress Free), 5 (Calm Child), 9 (HeadAid)
> Herbs and Foods: Chamomile, Lobelia, Calcium

Liver Invades Spleen:
> Herbal Categories: Regulate Chi, Tonify Chi (of
> Spleen)
> Formulas: 20 (HingaShtak), 12 (HepatoPure),
> Other Formulas: Minor Bupleurum
> Herbs and Foods: Dandelion Root; Green Vegetables,
> Apple Cider Vinegar and Honey, a teaspoon of each
> taken together before and/or after meals

Cold in Liver:
>Herbal Categories: Tonify Blood, Warm Interior
>Eliminate Cold, Vitalize Blood
>Formulas: 6 (Women's Treasure), 19 (Trikatu), 17
>(Herbal Uprising)
>Herbs and Foods: Ginger, Angelica, Cayenne,
>Prickly Ash bark

Kidney

Deficient Kidney Chi:
>Herbal Category: Tonify Chi
>Formulas: 25 (Tai Chi Ginseng Complex)
>Other Formulas: 36 (Wu Zi Wan)
>Herbs and Foods: Oxtail Soup, Pork Kidney, cooked
>food, Beans

Deficient Kidney Yang:
>Herbal Categories: Tonify Yang, Warm Interior
>Eliminate Cold
>Formulas: 28 (Yang Tonic), 19 (Trikatu)
>Other Formulas: 36 (Wu Zi Wan)
>Herbs and Foods: Oxtail Soup, Pork Kidney, Fenugreek
>seeds, Walnuts, Lamb, Beans, must eat all cooked food

Deficient Kidney Yin:
>Herbal Category: Tonify Yin
>Formulas: 27 (Yin Tonic)
>Herbs and Foods: Lean Pork, Pork Kidney, Seaweed,
>Oysters, Shellfish

Deficient Kidney Essence:
>Herbal Category: Tonify Yin (Kidney)
>Formulas: 27 (Yin Tonic), 18 (Vital Balance)
>Herbs and Foods: Black beans, Pork Kidney, Placenta

Pericardium

Invasion of Pericardium by Heat

Herbal Category: Clear Heat Purge Fire
Formulas: 14 (River of Life), 21 (Triphala)
Herbs and Foods: Violet, Hawthorne, Pansy Leaf

Small Intestine

Heat Being Transferred From the Heart to the Small Intestine
Herbal Categories: Clear Heat Purge Fire, Purge
Attack
Formulas: 14 (River of Life), 21 (Triphala)
Herbs and Foods: Violet, Hawthorne, Pansy Leaf

Large Intestine

Damp-Heat in the Large Intestine
Herbal Categories: Promote Water Flow Permeate
Wet, Purge-diuretic
Formulas: 21 (Triphala), 12 (HepatoPure), 13
(HerbaDerm)
Herbs and Foods: Poke Root, Cascara Sagrada Bark,
Rhubarb Root, Buckthorne Bark
Stasis of the Large Intestine
Herbal Categories: Purge-Attack, Purge-Lubricate
Formula: 21 (Triphala)
Herbs and Foods: Senna, Aloe, Cascara
Sagrada, Rhubarb, Buckthorn, Castor oil, Psyllium
Seeds, Flax Seeds

Stagnation of Blood and Heat in the Large Intestine
Herbal Categories: Regulate Chi, Vitalize Blood, Purge
Attack
Formulas: 21 (Triphala)
Herbs and Foods: Golden Seal, Rhubarb, Plums,
Stewed Prunes

Stomach

Retention of Food in the Stomach
Herbal Category: Remove Congestion

100

Formulas: 20 (HingaShtak)
Herbs and Foods: Radish Seed, Anise Seed, Asafoetida,
Fennel Seeds, Ginger

Retention of Fluid in the Stomach due to Cold
Herbal Categories: Fragrant Dissolve Wet, Promote
Water Flow, Permeate Wet, Warm Interior Eliminate
Cold, Purge Diuretic
Formulas: 20 (HingaShtak)
Other Formulas: 37 (Herbal Warmth)
Herbs and Foods: Fennel Seed, Anise Seed, Dill Seed,
Cardamom, Cloves

Gallbladder

Damp-Heat in the Gallbladder
Herbal Categories: Purge Attack, Purge Diuretic, Clear
Heat Dry Wet
Formulas: 12 (HepatoPure), 13 (HerbaDerm)
Herbs and Foods: Turmeric, Oregon Grape Root,
Goldenseal, Fringe Tree Bark, Dandelion

Urinary Bladder

Damp-Heat in the Urinary Bladder
Herbal Categories: clear heat, dry wet, promote water
flow
Formulas: 2 (Diurite)
Herbs and Foods: Uva Ursi, Gentian root, Pipsessewa,
Oregon grape, Barberry, Goldenseal, Aduki beans and
Mung Beans
Disturbance in the Function of the Urinary Bladder
Herbal Categories: Regulate Chi, Warm Interior and
eliminate coldness, Tonify yang
Formulas: 2 (Diurite), 17 (Herbal Uprising)
Other Formulas: 37 (Herbal Warmth)
Herbs and Foods: Juniper berries, Cinnamon, ginger,
Cubeb, Black pepper, Red pepper.

Part IV

20. Formulas

Their energetic conformation, indications and counter-indications

Upper Respiratory: Lungs, bronchioles and sinuses

Formula 1 (decongestant, relieves allergies and lungs)

Ma huang--- chief herb
Platycodon--- chief herb
Comfrey root--- assisting
Mullein--- assisting
Wild cherry bark--- assisting
Licorice--- assisting
Elecampane--- supporting
Ginger--- conducting
Cinnamon twigs--- conducting
Wild ginger root--- conducting

This formula is dispersing, decongesting, good for colds, flu, allergies, asthma and upper respiratory problems. It has a neutral to warm energy.

Dosage: Take two or more tablets, three or more times daily with warm water. It is excellent as a general treatment for smokers to help offset the harmful effects on the lungs.

Urinary Problems

Formula 2 (diuretic, removes damp stagnation)

Cleavers--- chief herb
Uva ursi--- chief herb
Poria--- chief herb
Dandelion root--- supporting
Marshmallow root--- assisting
Parsley root--- assisting
Ginger root--- conducting

This formula is dispersing, diuretic, harmonizes fluid metagolism, overcomes thirst, swelling, cystitis, and kidney weakness. It has a cool to neutral energy. Dosage: For general fluid balance and elimination take two or more tablets three times daily with warm water. For urinary inflammation take two tablets every two hours along with two Echinacea tablets.

Gallstones and Urinary Stones

Formula 3 (clears stones and damp heat of liver, gall and spleen)

Turmeric root--- chief herb
Gravel root--- chief herb
Parsley root--- chief herb
Dandelion root--- supporting
Marshmallow root--- assisting
Licorice--- assisting
Ginger root--- conducting

Having a cool energy, this formula is pain relieving, dispersing, detoxifying and diuretic. It relieves and helps dissolve pains of both gall and kidney and bladder stones. It can also treat diabetes by helping to regulate blood sugar.
Dosage: Take two tablets three times daily; for acute conditions take two tablets every two hours, tapering off as symptoms subside. Not recommended for pregnant women.

Prostate Formula

Formula 4 (tonifies male reproductive organ, clears prostate)

Saw Palmetto--- chief herb
Echinacea root--- assisting herb
Goldenseal--- assisting
Gravel root--- assisting
True Unicorn root--- assisting
Uva ursi--- assisting
Marshmallow root--- supporting
Cayenne--- conducting

This formula has a mild to neutral energy. It is detoxifying and dispersing, treats prostate problems of men, aids reproductive cycle and strengthens male potency.

Dosage: As a tonic, take two tablets three times daily. For acute conditions take every two hours tapering off as symptoms subside.

For Children

Formula 5 (calms mental anxiety, relieves surface tension for children)

Camomile--- chief herb
Catnip--- chief herb
Hawthorn berries--- supporting
Lemon balm--- chief herb
Semen Zizyphus--- chief herb
Gota Kola--- assisting
Pippli Pepper--- conducting
Licorice--- supporting
Dragon bone--- chief herb
Stevia--- supporting
Calcium Phosphate 6X, assisting
Kali Phos 6X, assisting
Mag Phos 6X, assisting

This formula has a cool energy. It is a soothing, calming, gentle and nourishing nerve tonic. Good for hyper-active children. It will also assist normal growth and development. Good for teething infants. It is available both in syrup and tablet form.

Dose: Take one or two tablets three times daily or as needed.

Gynecology

Formula 6 (regulates blood, hormones, menses, regulates female organs)

Dang quai--- chief herb
Lovage--- chief herb
False Unicorn--- chief herb
cooked Rehmannia--- chief herb
Cramp bark--- assisting

Paeonia alba--- assisting and conducting
Atractylodes alba--- assisting
Blue Cohosh--- assisting
Moutan--- supporting
Poria--- supporting
Ginger--- conducting

A blood tonic for women, this formula moves blood, regulates menstrual cycle for deficient blood and increases estrogen. It has a warm nature and is good for all menstrual disorders of women, ammenorrhea, menorrhagia, and dysmenorrhea. Specifically it is a more tonifying pre-ovulation formula while Formula 7 with Agnus Castus berries can be used for post ovulation. Oftentimes, the liver is responsible for most gynecological imbalances in women so that Formula 12 for the liver can also be taken with Formula 6. If there is accompanying fluid accumulation, the use of Diurite will also be very helpful. Generally, such an herbal program should be followed for a minimum of three months to achieve the kind of permanent results one may be seeking.

Dosage: As a tonic take 2 tablets three times daily. For acute conditions, take 2 tablets every two hours with warm water. This is not generally recommended for pregnant women.

Formula 7 (relieves menstrual problems, regulates energy, hormones)

Agnus castus--- chief herb
Dang quai--- assisting
Cramp bark--- assisting
Squaw vine--- chief herb
Cyperus--- supporting
Poria--- supporting
Ginger root--- 1 part.

For menstrual problems and regulating the female hormones. This formula with Agnus Castus regulates progesterone, helps regulate and smooth liver Chi, regulates Chi, calms the mind, increases B12, adds calcium, is a diuretic, clears the liver and neutralizes excess hormones. It is also good for cramps, PMS, moodiness and anxiety and has a more cooling energy. For difficult, chronic menstrual problems, alternate taking this formula after ovulation up to menstruation and Formula 6 after menstruation up to ovulation.

Dosage: As a tonic, take 2 tablets three times daily more or less as needed. For acute conditions, take more as above. Not generally recommended for pregnant women.

Stress and Nervous Tension

Formula 8 (calm mind, relieve nervous tension, sedate wind)

Valerian--- chief herb
Dragon bone--- chief herb
Oyster shell--- chief herb
Semen Zizyphus--- chief herb
Black Cohosh--- assisting
Camomile--- assisting
Hops--- assisting
Mistletoe (European)--- assisting
Skullcap--- chief herb
Wood Betony--- chief herb
Hawthorn berries--- supporting
Licorice--- supporting
American Ginseng--- supporting
Ginger--- conducting
    This formula has a mild, neutral and soothing energy and is tonic to the nerves. It relieves insomnia, general nervous tension, excessive irritability, anxiety and poor concentration.
    Dosage: As a tonic, take 2 tablets three times daily. For acute conditions, take two tablets every two hours. Not recommended for pregnant women.

Formula 9 (relieve head congestion, pain)

Feverfew--- chief herb
Semen Viticis--- chief herb
Notopterygium root---chief herb
Ligusticum--- chief herb
Angelica--- chief herb
Licorice--- supporting
Sileris--- assisting
Cyperus--- assisting
Schizonepeta--- conducting
Tea--- conducting

This formula relieves nervousness, headache, colds and flu. It has a warm energy.

Dosage: Take one or two tablets with boiled warm water every two hours or as needed. Contraindicated for pregnant women.

Heart and Mind

Formula 10 (nourish heart Chi, blood, regulate circulation, calm mind)

Hawthorn berries--- chief herb
Tienchi Ginseng--- assisting and conducting
Motherwort--- assisting and conducting
Dang quai--- assisting
Salvia milthiorrhiza--- chief herb and conducting
Polygala--- assisting and conducting
Borage--- supporting
Juniper berries--- supporting
Codonopsis--- supporting
Longan berries--- supporting

For the heart and spirit, this formula calms the mind from excessive thoughts, nourishes Blood and Yin and assists circulation. It has a warm circulating energy and is useful for arteriosclerosis, restlessness, low energy, palpitations and heart pains and most heart problems.

Dosage: As a tonic, take 2 tablets three times daily. For acute conditions, take more as needed. Not recommended for pregnant women.

Weight Control

Formula 11 (detoxify blood and lymphatic system, reduce fat)

Triphala--- chief herb
Spirulina--- chief herb
Kelp--- chief herb
Cleavers--- chief herb
Fennel--- conducting
Cascara--- assisting
Chaparral--- assisting

Echinacea--- assisting
Ginger--- conducting
Gambir--- assisting
Rhubarb--- assisting
Watercress--- assisting
Atractylodes--- assisting
Stephania--- assisting
Licorice--- supporting
Astragalus--- chief herb
Ma huang--- assisting
Semen Zizyphus--- assisting
Mustard seed--- assisting

Good for opening gently opening all the channels of elimination and detoxification in a balanced way. It will aid assimilation and therefore further help satiate hunger. It has a slightly cool, dispersing energy and is good for general detoxification and weight reduction.

Dosage: 2 to 4 tablets three times daily. It is excellent to take with a diet of warm soya milk for weight reduction or a tea of cleavers and fennel seed combined.

Liver

Formula 12 (detoxify liver, blood, regulate liver Chi)

Bupleurum--- chief, assisting and conducting
Milk thistle seeds--- chief and assisting
Cyperus--- conducting
Dandelion root--- chief herb
Oregon Grape root--- chief herb
Wild Yam root--- assisting
Angelica--- assisting
Lycii berries--- supporting
Fennel seed--- conducting
Ginger--- conducting
Green Citrus peel--- conducting

A relatively balanced energy, this formula regulates Liver metabolism and dredges and detoxifies the Liver while supporting Liver Yin (Blood). It is useful for hepatitis, chest pains, colitis due to liver irregularities, constipation, cirrhoses, gynecology, and general blood detoxification. Unlike many other cholagogues, it also helps tonify Liver Blood so it is especially good for Deficient conditions with Blood and Yin Deficiency. Dose: 2 tablets three times daily with warm water.

Skin and Genital Herpes

Formula 13 (detoxify blood and lymph system, reduce heat, clear skin)

Echinacea--- chief herb
Yellow Dock--- chief herb
Gentian root--- chief herb
Golden Seal--- chief herb
Myrrh gum--- conducting
Bupleurum--- chief and assisting
Poria--- assisting
Wild Yam root--- supporting
Marshmallow root--- supporting

This formula has a cool energy and is detoxifying. It disperses Damp Heat from the lower warmer (the pelvic cavity) making it useful for acute and chronic venereal diseases including herpes, Pelvic inflammatory disease, leucorrhea, gonorrhea, syphilis, general skin eruptions. It is good for blood purification and helping to resolve inflammation and pus.
Dosage: 2 to 4 tablets three times daily with warm water. Patients should be warned against the use of all stimulants including drugs, alcohol, coffee, sugar and acidic foods such as tomatoes and citrus.

Blood Purification, Skin and Inflammatory Conditions

Formula 14 (detoxify blood, clear heat)

Echinacea root--- chief herb
Golden seal ---- chief herb
chaparral ------ chief herb
Honeysuckle flowers---- chief herb
Forsythia blossoms--- chief herb
Sarsaparilla root--- chief herb
Yellow dock root--- chief herb

109

American ginseng--- supporting herb
Ginger root --- conducting herb
Cinnamon twigs --- conducting herb

This blood purifying formula has a cool detoxifying energy. It is useful for inflammatory conditions, skin eruptions, fevers, toxicity of blood and lymph, boils, sores and cancer. It can be used for both bacterial and viral infections. For the treatment of flu, take four tablets with warm water two or three times a day.

Dosage: Two to four tablets taken three times daily with warm water. Diet should be simple, avoiding heating and dispersing foods including denatured foods, drugs, stimulants, peppers, sugar (including fruit juices, and fruits), alcohol and excess meat.

Chronic Degenerative Diseases, Tumors, Cancers and Cysts

Formula 15 (clear blood, lymph, resolve Tumors)

Pau d'Arco--- Chief herb
Echinacea root--- chief herb
Chaparral--- chief herb
Red clover blossoms--- chief herb
Poria--- assisting herb
Grifola--- assisting herb
American ginseng--- assisting herb
Kelp--- assisting and conducting herb

Cool natured and dispersing, this formula is a mild diuretic, helping to resolve tumors, cysts and lymphatic congestion. It is specifically useful for chronic degenerative diseases such as cancer, but good for other chronic conditions as well. It is ideal to take along with DEFENSE FORCE for patients undergoing chemo or radiation therapy to help offset some of the negative side effects. This formula can be combined with good results with the River of Life formula.

Dosage: Two to four tablets three times daily with warm water or red clover tea.

Immune System

Formula 16 (strengthen wei Chi, prevent sickness)

Pau d' Arco--- chief herb
Echinacea root--- chief herb
Astragalus--- chief herb
Schizandra berries--- assisting herb
Ligustrum fruit--- assisting herb
Chaparral--- assisting herb
Golden seal--- assisting herb
Garlic--- conducting herb
Ginger root--- conducting herb

Tonifies both Yin and Yang as it clears deficient heat, protecting the righteous energy or the immune system. It is to be considered in the prevention and treatment of the immune system, general weakness, colds, flu, candida albicans yeast overgrowth, cancer, AIDS and immune Deficiency diseases generally.

Dose: For prevention take two tablets once or twice daily. For treatment 2 tablets three times daily with warm water or mild licorice tea.

Natural Antibiotic, Blood and Lymphatic Cleanser

Echinacea Extract (clear heat)

Pure extracted Echinacea Angustifolia, E. Palida and E. Purpurea.

Cool and detoxifying, this formula counteracts all inflammatory conditions of a solid or Excess nature. It is only useful as an adjunctive for Deficiency Heat conditions. Echinacea tonifies the surface immune system, aiding the process of anti-body production. It can be used as an herbal antibiotic alone or in combination with Formula 15.

Dosage: Acute: take 2 tablets at least every two hours, tapering off as symptoms subside. Continue taking three times daily for a week or two after all symptoms have disappeared. If there is no improvement within the first three days, the inflammation is usually due to a Deficient condition, in which case, combine it with a small amount of ginseng.

Circulation and Warmth

Formula 17 (warming, stimulant, relieve congestion)

Ginger root--- chief
Cinnamon twigs--- chief
Cayenne--- chief
WHITE-PINE bark--- assisting
Cloves--- assisting
Bayberry bark--- assisting
Marsh mallowroot--- harmonizing
Licorice root--- harmonizing

This formula has a warm, dispersing, and drying energy. It is similar to the renowned Composition Powder of early American herbal medical practice. It is a very useful herbal first aid remedy for treating the first stages of colds, flu, congestion, overeating, bloatedness, diarrhea and stagnant circulatory conditions. It may also be used for stimulating hot foot and tub baths for any of the above. Mostly used as an acute remedy for occasional use, it is not recommended for those having chronic inflammatory conditions with Deficient Heat.

Dosage: Take three to four tablets with warm water or ginger and honey tea at the first sign of cold or flu. Repeat as needed.

Glandular Formula

Formula 18 (harmonize and regulate hormones)

Dang quai--- chief and conducting
American Ginseng--- chief
Saw Palmetto berries--- chief
Agnus castus--- chief
Kelp--- chief
Sarsaparilla--- assisting
Black Cohosh--- assisting
Golden seal--- assisting
Licorice--- harmonizing

Ginger--- conducting

This formula has a neutral to warm energy, is a general glandular tonic, counteracts aging, preserves youthfulness, is good for pubescent children and retarded growth, menopause, strengthens hormone function, tonifies both Yin and Yang and counteracts impotency and frigidity.

Dosage: As a tonic take two to four tablets two or three times daily.

AYURVEDIC FORMULAS

Rasayanas

Rasayanas represent a special branch of Ayurvedic medicine which is literally involved in the process of rejuvenation and revitalization. There area number of extremely valuable and key rasayanas of which some of the most important are described below.

Mucus, Allergies, Digestion

Formula 19 (trikatu)
Equal parts Ginger root, Piper nigrum, Bibo (Piper longum), Honey.

This formula has a hot, spicy energy and is dispersing and drying for Damp conditions. It helps overcomes mucus, making it very useful for allergies, treats colds, helps reduce fat, aids digestion and circulation and warms internally. A specific remedy for clear Damp discharges that often occur in cold, damp climates, it should be taken by nearly everyone living in such environments and then suspended during the warm summer months.

Dosage: Take one or two tablets three times a day. Patient should be advised to reduce intake of dairy, fruits and juices.

Formula 20 (Hinga Shtak)

Atractylodes alba--- chief herb
Caraway seed--- chief herb
Cumin seed--- chief herb

113

Dandelion--- assisting herb
Ginger--- conducting and chief herb
Piper nigrum--- conducting herb
Slippery Elm--- assisting herb
Asafoetida--- chief herb
Bibo (Piper longum)--- conducting herb
Citrus peel--- conducting herb
Rock salt--- supporting herb

Having a warm energy, this formula regulates Chi, aids digestion counteracts acidity, digestive weakness, eliminates gas, bloating, and is one of the best formulas to use for hypoglycemia and the symptoms associated with candida albicans yeast overgrowth. It can be powdered and added to food when eating to enhance digestion or taken either before or after meals with warm water.

Formula 21 (Triphala) (reduce excess, regulate digestion and elimination)
Equal parts Emblica officinalis, Terminalia belerica, and two parts Terminalia chebulae.

Triphala ("tri' = three; "phala" = fruits), consists of the combination of the fruit of the chebulic, beleric and emblic myrobalan trees respectively. These are popularly known in India as Harad, Behada and Amla respectively. Triphala is widely regarded as a purgative and laxative but in fact it is considered a Rasayana and rejuvenator. Its special value, therefore, is both as a regulator of elimination as well as a rejuvenator of the whole body.

Harada and Behada has a hot energy, while Amla is cool. This means that Triphala being a combination of all three is quite balanced, making it useful as an internal cleansing, detoxifying formula for everyone including more sensitive type individuals as well as vegetarians.

Regular, daily use of Triphala will promote normal appetite, good digestion, the increase of red blood cells and haemoglobin and the removal of undesirable fat. Triphala will also eliminate what is called deficient heat in Chinese medicine. This is a feeling of heat and burning on the chest, legs, palms and/or soles of the feet all representing a B vitamin deficiency in Western medicine. Triphala taken regularly will promote the absorption and utilization of the B vitamins and will have the symptoms of deficient heat described completely relieved.

Of primary importance is the use of Triphala as a bowel regulator for which it is considered as safe as food and non-habit forming, even on a daily basis. There is no wonder that in India there is a saying amongst the people comparing the importance of Triphala to that of a mother.

Since Triphala is a tonic, cleanser and blood purifier, there is still one other important use for it and that is as a strengthener of the eyes. Triphala can be taken as an eyewash daily and will strengthen the vision, counteract many eye defects and eliminate redness and soreness.

Dose: As a blood purifier, reducing and cleansing agent, take two tablets three times daily. As an occasional tonic laxative, take 2 to 6 tablets in the evening with a cup of boiled water. For eye problems, crush two tablets and steep in a half cup of boiling water, cool, strain and use as an eyewash.

Bulk Nutrient Laxative

Formula 22.(Triphala-Three Seeds Combination)

Equal parts psyllium, flax, chia seeds, with triphala, wild yam root, anise seed, ginger, yellow citrus peel, and Stevia rebaudiana.

One or two teaspoons stirred into a 6 oz. glass of water or diluted fruit juice. Drink immediately for optimum palatibility. Children should take less according to age.

Formula 23 (Chyavanprash) (tonify wei Chi, prevent sickness, revitalize energy)

One of the most potent and delicious tonics known! In Ayurveda it is considered a Rasayana, which is a preparation that is use for rejuvenation and revitalization. "Chyavan" was the name of a great sage who first created the formula. The legend was that the daughter of a famous emperor was innocently playing, blindfolded in the forest when she accidentally stumbled upon the famous saint in the practice of his austerities. Not knowing who it was or what she was doing, she innocently ran her fingers through his hair and garlanded him with flowers. Her father, the emperor, came upon her so doing and thus requested the sage to marry his daughter as it was the custom in India that a woman could have only one man in her life. The aged sage requested some time to prepare for the marriage. During this time he created Chyavanprash and remained on it for two months to regain his youthful vitality and virility. He was then able to marry the young girl and share conjugal bliss with his young wife.

Chyavanprash is made only with selected and fresh Indian Gooseberries, called Amla or Amlakis (Emblic myrobalans). These fruits are considered the major health food herb throughout India. They are the highest known source of easily assimilable vitamin C but of equal importance, the vitamin C in amla is bound up with certain harmless tannins which allow the fruits to maintain their potency of vitamin C content even after drying or subjecting them to heat. Normally, vitamin C is quickly dissipated under such conditions but not so with amla.

Hundreds of fresh amla fruits go into the making of Chyavanprash. They are first cleaned, washed and tied in a cloth and boiled in water slowly down to 1/6 the amount. The decoction is then strained and the seeds are removed and discarded. The remains of the amla fruit are then fried in sesame oil and butter and reduced to a paste. The paste is combined with the strained decoction and further boiled and reduced with jaggury, (crude brown sugar with molasses). At this point approximately 34 to 50 herbs, depending upon the version of Chyavanprash used, is added in powder form. When the preparation is well cooked honey is added to complete the process of manufacture.

Chyavanprash is celebrated throughout India and is as well known and honored tonic by the Indians as the famous ginseng is by the Chinese. The ancient Sanskrit texts state how it can be regularly used by the old and debilitated, also for chronic bronchitis, allergies, immune weakness, feverishness, debility, emaciation, chronic cardiac disorders, gout, disorders of the urinary tract, impotence, infertility, by the young infant, the very old, debilitated and very thin. Being both nourishing and nutritious, it will increase longevity, mental alertness, and glowing complexion. It will clarify the urine and bring regularity of evacuation. It will first remove parasites and toxins and then set about curing anorexia, indigestion and dyspepsia when taken over a prolonged period. Finally, regular use of

Chyavanprash will induce sexual strength and vigor in a man to help satisfy a woman.

Many varieties of commercial Chyavanprash are made with excess sugar or white sugar which diminishes its value. Besides amla, the herbs used in Chyavanpraṣh have diuretic, carminative, mildly laxative and tonic properties. They improve circulation, counteract coughs, expectorate phlegm, and tone up the entire system. Some varieties will have added musk for virility, saffron to stimulate circulation, iron, gold, amber, silver or other purified metalic oxides that can augment the virtues of Chyavanprash.

Half to one teaspoon taken each morning followed by warm water, herb tea or warm milk will treat low blood sugar, anemia, dyspepsia, build up the tissues and cells of the body and strengthen the vital organs of the heart, liver, kidneys and sense organs of both the young and old. Chyavanprash, as an herbal preparation, is truly the king of the herb foods.

Formula 24 (guggul) (clears channels, relieves pains, stiffness)

Guggula is made from the resin of "Balsamodendron Mukul"; Sanscrit, guggula; English, Salaitree, gum guggal or Indian Bedellium. It is very closely related to myrrh gum for which many books describe its use interchangeably. When fresh, it is moist, viscid and fragrant with a golden color. It will melt in the sun and emulsify in hot water.

Guggula is considered to be anti-kapha or mucus and as such reduces fat. Since it is also oily, it will alleviate disorders of the nervous system. Being mild in nature, only prolonged, long term usage will cause it to aggravate pitta or fire. Most importantly, it is considered the most potent remedy against "Ama" which is an accumulation of cholesterol, thickened mucus and other materials associated with the aging process and cause various circulatory problems including arteriosclerosis, arthritis, rheumatism, heart problems, high blood pressure, obesity, enlargement of the prostate and all other diseases associated with aging.

It is widely known and celebrated throughout India and freely recommended by Ayurvedic doctors for all diseases associated with arthritis, rheumatism, sciatica, back and joint pains.

Guggula is often combined with Triphala to make Triphala guggula. This is taken morning and evening to counteract obesity, blood disorders, constipation, skin problems, chronic venereal disease, ascites, sores that are difficult to heal and all such diseases associated with an accumulation of Ama which gradually inhibits the natural rejuvenative processes of the body.

Guggula is made according to a traditional method of wrapping the resin in a porous natural fibre cloth and boiling it in a decoction of Triphala to purify the resins so they can easily pass through the system without causing any toxicity. The guggul decoction is then further cooked down to a thick paste and spread out on a suitable pan or holder to dry in the sun. This can then be broken into chunks or powdered for use as Guggul.

Yoga Raj Guggula is the most well known preparation of Guggul in India. It is used for many disorders including sciatica, rheumatism, gout, arthritis, amenorrhea, obesity, painful menses in women or stopped menstruation, hemorrhoids, worms, fistula and impotence. It is a rejuvenator and by purifying the blood promoting normal circulation allays pain. It will increase elimination of waste through sweat, promotes normal secretion of digestive juices, regulate the bowels as well as prevent and eliminate intestinal gases. It has deep, lasting normalizing effect upon the female menstrual flow; where there is excess, it will decrease and where it is blocked, promote it. Finally, Guggula is an excellent circulatory tonic to take to promote flexibility, internal strength and stamina, making it very useful for athletes.

When combined with Ashwagandha and Turmeric, guggul is one of the most effective anti-arthritic compounds. It will eliminate body stiffness, aches and pains and restore youthful flexibility.

Dose: about 250 to 500 Ml. are taken twice daily.

Formula 25 (shilajita) (tonifies kidneys, counteracts deficiencies)

This is the natural exudate of certain rocks and stones found in the Himalayas. It very much resembles and smells like asphalt which is the English name for it. In its natural state, Shilajit is eaten by rats and monkeys. It is considered to be the

118

urinary tonic par excellence in Ayurveda, being a dark black color, it also corresponds to the black colored herbs such as rehmannia root, which are considered kidney-adrenal tonics in Chinese medicine. Shilajit is obtained by pulverizing the stones and boiling them in water. The stones used are black and greasy looking. After the boiling, a creamy film develops and this is removed and dried in the sun. To purify, Shilajit, and thus aid their assimilability, the stones are boiled in a decoction of Triphala.

Shilajit is naturally high in iron and other valuable minerals making it very useful for all wasting, degenerative diseases especially diseases such as diabetes, chronic urinary tract problems, impotence, infertility and to promote strong bones, the healing of fractures, osteoarthritis, spondylosis and so forth.

It is well known for its anti-diabetic properties, reducing blood sugar and diabetes in the early stages.

Normally Shilajit is found as a a paste preparation and it is dissolved in a little boiled hot water or hot milk and taken twice daily.

CHINESE FORMULAS

Formula 26 (tonify spleen Yang, vitalize energy)

Panax Ginseng--- chief herb
American Ginseng--- chief herb
Siberian Ginseng--- chief and conducting herb
Codonopsis --- chief herb
Tienchi Ginseng--- chief and conducting
Atractylodes alba--- chief and assisting
Polygonum multiflorum--- supporting
Astragalus mongolicus--- chief herb
Dang quai--- assisting and conducting
Poria--- supporting
Ginger--- conducting
Licorice--- supporting

Tonifies spleen Chi, Yang and Blood, thus it has a warm, strengthening energy. It is useful for low energy, fatigue, hypoglycemia, forgetfulness, lowered immune system, and builds energy gradually over a long period of time.

119

Dosage: For extreme Deficient conditions, simmer four tablets in 3 cups of water and add some meat, grains, root vegetables, to make a soup. Can be taken two or three times daily by those with Deficiency and Coldness. It can be taken each morning as an herbal energy pill to help maintain energy and youthful vitality.

Formula 27 (Shujin San) (promote circulation of Blood and Chi, counteract spasms)

Dang quai--- chief
Ligusticum--- chief
Achryanthes--- chief
Lycii berries--- assisting
Gambir--- assisting
Sileris--- assisting
Angelica Tu huo--- chief, assisting, conducting
Dipsacus--- chief
Chaenomeles--- chief
Tienchi Ginseng--- chief, assisting, conducting
Noptopterygium--- chief, assisting

A tonic for the kidneys and liver, this formula soothes muscles and tendons, increases general body flexibility, improves blood circulation, relieves aches and pains, arthritis, gout, rheumatism, pain of lower back and legs, numbness and dyskinesia.

Dosage: Can be taken either as a tablet or alcoholic based extract (which is particularly useful for the aged with circulatory problems). As a tincture, take 30 drops two or three times a day. As tablets, take 2 two or three times a day.

Formula 28 (Yin) (nourishing, tonify Fluids and body substance)

Rehmannia (cooked)--- chief
Cornus berries--- assisting
Moutan Peony--- assisting
Poria--- assisting
Dioscorea--- supporting
Alisma--- assisting
Lycii berries--- chief

Chrysanthemum flowers--- chief, assisting
Polygonum multiflorum--- chief, assisting, supporting
Ligustrum :lucidi--- chief
Saw palmetto berries--- assisting, supporting

A Yin tonic having a nourishing a neutral, cool energy. Tonifying, kidney Yin, strengthens weak kidney urinary function and is useful for the treatment of impotence, ringing ears, aching lower back and knees, nightsweats, diabetes and involuntary emission. It is also good for night blindness, photophobia, vision weakness, hypertension and regenerating the liver. Supporting the cooling aspect of the adrenal hormones, it might be considered as increasing feelings of love and compassion. A good tonic for those over the age of 40.

Dosage: Take two tablets two or three times a day with warm water, a little miso, tamari sauce or a pinch of salt.

Formula 29 (Yang) (tonify adrenals, hormones, vital energy)

Rehmannia (cooked)--- chief
Withania somnifera--- chief, supporting
Cornus berries--- chief
Moutan Peony--- assisting, supporting
Poria--- chief, assisting
Dioscorea--- supporting
Alisma--- assisting
Psoralea bean--- assisting
Cuscutae seed--- chief
Cistanches--- chief
Morindae--- chief
Epimedium--- chief
Saw palmetto berries--- assisting, chief
Schizandra berries--- supporting
Lycii berries--- supporting
Dang Quai--- supporting, conducting
Aconitum praeparata--- chief, conducting
Cinnamon bark--- chief, conducting

Having a very warm nature, this formula tonifies kidney Yang. It strengthens weak adrenal function and is useful in the treatment of general coldness, impotence, chronic nephritis, kidney atrophy, edema, difficult urination, chronic cystitis, diabetes, lower back pains, painful joints and cold, deficient constipation. It increases drive and motivation. Another useful longevity tonic for those past the age of 40.

Dosage: Take 2 tablets two or three times a day with warm water with a little miso, tamari sauce or a pinch of salt.

Formula 30 (Pueraria Combination) (Ko Ken Tang or Kuzu Root Tea) (relieve surface, relax muscles, promote diaphoretics)

Pueraria root--- chief
Ma huang--- chief, conducting
Cinnamon twigs--- chief, conducting
Peony alba--- assisting
Jujube date--- supporting
Licorice--- supporting
Ginger--- assisting, conducting

This warm natured formula is generally useful for all constitutional types for the treatment of colds, flu, pneumonia, bronchitis, upper shoulder and muscle tightness and soreness, coughs and gastrointestinal diseases.

Formula 31 (Minor Bupleurum Combination) (Hsiao chai hu tang) (relieve diseases that are half internal and half superficial, half weak, half strong)

Bupleurum--- chief
Scutellaria root--- assisting
Pinellia--- assisting
Ginseng--- supporting
Jujube date --- supporting
Licorice--- supporting
Ginger--- supporting, conducting

This is a general formula for prolonged symptoms of cold, flu, asthma, pneumonia, bronchitis, headaches, nasal congestion, shoulder stiffness, tuberculosis and pleurisy. It is also good for hypoglycemia and hepatitis, and for diseases that are half acute and half chronic, half weak and half strong, half Internal and half External, half Yin and half Yang. This is one of the most commonly indicated formulas and can be taken over a prolonged period for promoting general health.

CHINESE TONIC HERB FOODS

Chinese tonic herb foods are a uniquely different and delicious way to take Chinese herbs. Finely powdered herbs are specially heated and mixed with honey and ghee which aid their assimilation into the cells and tissues of the body. Herbs are popularly taken in this way in China and India because individuals with a more Yin-Damp condition (such as most vegetarians might have), are not recommended to take too much fluids (including herb teas).

Formula 32 (Jade Screen) (Yipingfeng San) (For Internal Coldness)

Astragalus--- chief
Atractylodes alba--- chief
Sileris--- assisting, conducting

This Chinese herb food is for the immune system and Internal Coldness. Tonifying the immune system, it protects one's self from sickness. It energizes and warms all the Internal vital organs, strengthens the Chi of protection (Wei Chi) and is good for general poor health with frequent colds, flus and a tendency to sickness, perspiration from weakness and poor health. It is a delicious tonic suitable for young and old and is generally safe to take year round on a regular basis. Remember that most warm natured tonics are not taken during active acute inflammatory conditions unless specially prescribed.
Dosage: One half to one teaspoon once or twice daily.

Formula 33 (Si Wu Tang) (Tonify Blood)

Dang quai--- chief, conducting
Rehmannia (cooked) --- Chief
Peony alba--- Assisting, conducting
Ligusticum wallichii--- assisting, conducting

Tonifies blood, counteracts anemia, regulates menstruation, good for irregular menstruation in women. Dose: one teaspoon two or three times daily.

123

Formula 34 (Four nobles) (Si Junza Tang) (Tonify spleen Chi)

Ginseng---chief
Codonopsis--- chief
Atractylodes--- chief
Poria---assisting
Licorice--- harmonizing

Strengthens the Chi, aids digestion, tonifies the spleen Chi, strengthens the spleen-pancreas and stomach, counteracts weakness and fatigue.
Dose: one teaspoon two or three times daily.

Formula 35 (Gui Pi Tang) (Tonify spleen and heart, helps control mind)

Codonopsis---chief
Dang quai--- chief
Astragalus--- assisting
Atractylodes--- chief
Poria--- chief
Saussurea--- assisting, conducting
Longan berries--- supporting
Jujube dates--- supporting
Zizyphus seeds--- chief, assisting
Polygala root--- chief, assisting
Licorice root--- supporting

Tonifies Chi, centers the mind, strengthens spleen Chi, aids digestion, calming, helps insomnia, palpitations, asthenia, weak heart, poor appetite. Dose: one teaspoon 2 or 3 times daily.

Formula 36 (Eight Precious Herbs) (Ba Zhen Wan) (tonifies Chi and Blood)

Codonopsis--- chief
Dang quai--- chief
Ligusticum--- chief, assisting
Atractylodes--- chief, assisting
Peony alba--- assisting, conducting
Licorice--- supporting

Poria--- assisting
Rehmannia (cooked)--- chief

This Chinese herb food is a tonic for Blood and Energy. Take as an overall tonic and also for specific conditions such as anorexia, anemia and weakness.
Dosage: One half to one teaspoon is eaten once or twice daily.

Formula 37 (Wu Zi Wan) (tonifies both kidney-adrenal Yin and Yang)

Semen Plantago--- chief, assisting
Poria--- chief, assisting
Alisma--- chief
Rehmannia (cooked)--- chief
Dioscorea--- assisting, supporting
Semen Cuscutae--- chief
Lycii berries--- chief
Schizandra berries--- chief
Fructus Rubi (Raspberry)--- assisting
Cornus berries--- chief

A kidney-adrenal tonic good for both kidney Yin and Yang. It is good for supporting the adrenals, improving health and longevity. Amongst other things, it can be used for urinary weakness and improving general health, hair, complexion and counteracting impotence.
Dosage: Take one half to one teaspoon once or twice daily. For those over the age of forty it is best taken with a tablespoon or so of rice wine once or twice daily.

Formula 38 (tonify Yang, increase warmth)

Cinnamon bark--- chief
Ginger root--- chief
Atractylodes alba--- chief, assisting
Aconitum praeparata--- chief

Raises body metabolism, promotes circulation and diges- tion as it warms the whole body. Being a hot natured formula, it is good in the winter and for all Yin conditions associated with coldness, clear allergic discharges, clear urine, loose stool, weak digestion, low energy and palor and chronic bronchitis. Do not give for excess Yang-Heat or wasting Heat (Yin Deficient) conditions.

Dosage: Take one-eighth to one-quarter teaspoon once to three times daily.

Formula 39 (Bu Zhong Yi Chi Wan) (Formula for maximum Chi tonification)

Astragalus--- chief
Ginseng--- chief
Atractylodes--- chief, assisting
Licorice--- supporting
Dang Quai--- assisting, supporting, conducting
Cimicifuga--- conducting
Bupleurum--- conducting, assisting
Citrus peel--- assisting
Jujube date--- supporting
Ginger--- assisting, conducting

The formula for maximum tonification, chronic weakness, T.B., gastropsis, anorexia, abdominal distension, loss of weight during the summer, neuresthenia, impotence, uterine prolapse, hemorrhoids, rectal prolapse, monoplegia, ephidrosis, hernia, chronic gonorrhea, diarrhea, malaria, suppuration and hemorrhage. The individual will have a weak pulse, with general fatigue, mild fever, night sweats, headache, weak digestion, and palpitations at the umbilicus.

Dose: 1/2 to 1 teaspoon two or three times daily as a milder tonic, one can take 1/4 to 1/2 a teaspoon twice a day.

Single Herb Formulas and Classifications:

Emotional Balance (Agnus Castus) used to regulate chi, treats PMS and post menopausal syndromes.

St. Johnswort (Hypericum Perforatum) used to calm liver wind, relieve nerve pains, clear heat especially of viral infections.

Ginkgo Leaf extract (Ginkgo Biloba) used to promote blood circulation both generally and of the head and brain, treats tinnitus, senile dementia, Alzheimer's disease, chronic circulatory problems.

Suma (Pfaffia paniculata) Called "Brazilian Ginseng", it is used to tonify chi, especially spleen chi and yang, it is used in Brazil for many chronic diseases including chronic fatigue syndrome, diabetes, cancer, arthritis, digestive weakness and impotence.

Siberian Ginseng (Eleutherococus senticosus) used as a chi tonic and to increase the body's resistance to stress.

Valerian Root Extract (Valeriana officinalis) used for insomnia, nervousness, anxiety and pain.

Some important keys to herbal healing

Formulas are used according to functions rather then diseases. Herbs often work better when used in formula because they can be made to enhance the primary actions of each other (chief herbs), assisting the actions of the primary (chief) herbs, conduct and focus the main therapeutic action of the primary (chief) herbs, support the Energy, Blood, body Essence as needed to maximize the healing strategy of the primary herbs.

Thus formulas can be put together according to the heating or cooling properties of individual herbs, the tonifying or eliminating properties, the upward, downward, inward or outward direction of specific herbs, to counterbalance undesirable effects in other herbs.

Often, it is more effective to use a combination of formulas together rather then a single one. The body is complex. Disease most often arises out of a multiplicity of causes and imbalances and therefore require more complicated treatment using several formulas with clearly targeted functions such as elimination, reducing, tonification, harmonizing, purging, and so forth.

Herbs possess not only specific micronutrients in easily assimilable abundance but they enhance the body's ability to better assimilate and utilize those nutrients which makes them superior to other types of supplements. Further, unlike most vitamin and mineral supplements, herbs are all organically derived directly from nature.

Some herbal formulas such as formulas number 11, 12, 13, 14, 15, 21 are eliminative in nature; others such as numbers 1, 5, 6, 7, 8, 9, 18, 20, 23, 26 are regulating; still others such as 6, 10, 16, 22, 24, 25, 27, 28, 31, 32, 33,34, 35, 36, 38 are nourishing and tonifying.

Planetary Formulas

1. Breeze free
2. Diurite
3. Stone Free
4. Witasu
5. Calm Child
6. Women's Treasure
7. Women's Comfort
8. Stress Free
9. HeadAid
10. Life Pulse
11. Triphala Herbal Diet
12. HepatoPure
13. HerbaDerm
14. River of Life
15. Complete Pau d'Arco Program
16. Immune Force
17. Herbal Uprising
18. Vital Balance
19. Trikatu
20. HingaShtak
21. Triphala
22. Tri-Cleanse
23. Chyavanprash
24. Guggula
25. Shilajit
26. Tai Chi
27. Flexibility tonic
28. Yin Energetics
29. Yang Energetics
30. Pueraria Combination
31. Minor Bupleurum Combination
32. Jade Screen
33. Si Wu Tang
34. Si Junza Tang
35. Gui Pi Tang
36. Eight Precious Herbs
37. Wu Zi Wan
38. Herbal Warmth
39. Elixir of Life

BIBLIOGRAPHY

A Barefoot Doctor's Manual, Seattle: ts
Cloudburst Press, 1977
Beijing, Shanghai, Nanjing Colleges of Traditional Chinese
Medicine and The Acupuncture Institute of the Academy of
Traditional Chinese Medicine.

Essentials of Chinese Acupuncture, Beijing: Foreign Lan-
guages Press, 1980

Felter and Lloyd, King's American Dispensatory, Portland,
Oregon: Eclectic Medical Publications, 1983

Kaptchuk, Ted J., The Web That Has No Weaver, New York,
N.Y.: Congdon & Weed, Inc., 1983

Kushi, Michio, The Book of Macrobiotics, Elmsford, New
York: Japan Publications, 1977

Lad, Vasant, Ayurveda, The Science of Self-Healing, Santa Fe,
New Mexico: Lotus Press, 1984

Muramoto, Naboru, Healing Ourselves, New York, NY: Avon
Books, 1973

Shanghai College of Traditional Medicine, Acupuncture, A
Comprehensive Text, Chicago, Il: Eastland Press, 1981

Tierra, Michael, Planetary Herbology, publ. by Lotus Press,
Santa Fe, New Mexico, 1988.

Tierra, Michael, The Way of Herbs, New York, N.Y.: Pocket
Books (Simon & Schuster), 1980

Where to Purchase Herbs and Planetary Formulas: Call or
write Threshold Distributing, 23 Janis Way, Scotts Valley, Ca.
95066, 1-800-468-7410 or 408-438-1700

Biography

Michael Tierra is a California State certified acupuncture doctor and is the recipient of a degree in Doctor of Oriental Medicine from San Francisco College of Acupuncture. He is the author of a milestone book, Way of Herbs (published by Simon and Schuster) integrating Western herbs and nutrition with the oriental principles of energetic diagnostics, The Art of Planetary Herbology, his latest book categorizing Western herbs according to the Chinese classification system (published by Lotus Press), and The Herbal Tarot (with Candice Cantin - published by U.S. Games). He, along with his wife Lesley Tierra, is also the author of the East West Herbal Correspondence Course. Michael and his wife conduct a busy clinical schedule in Santa Cruz, Ca., where they can be reached for professional consultation.

Being devoted to both native North American herbology as well as traditional Chinese and East Indian Ayurvedic medicines, Michael's major focus has been to begin the process of integrating the profound healing wisdom of the East into Western herbology and to encourage the use of native North American herbs into the practice of Chinese herbology. This integration of East and West he calls Planetary Herbology.

To demonstrate the effectiveness of this integrated concept, he has formulated Planetary Herbal Products which are available and sold in health food stores throughout the country as well as widely used professionally.

Lesley Tierra is a California State and Nationally certified acupuncturist. She has a practice in Santa Cruz, California, with her husband where she combines acupuncture, herbs and food therapies.

She collaborated with Michael to produce the East West Herbal Correspondence Course, a self-paced home study course in the principles of Chinese, Western and Ayurvedic diagnosis and herbology and her own Children's Herbal.

Lesley has taught herbs and nutrition at Twin Lakes College in Santa Cruz, herbology and shiatsu massage at the Santa Cruz Wholistic Health Center, and herbs and nutrition with Michael Tierra at Heartwood College (Santa Cruz). She currently teaches Chinese Planetary Herbal Diagnosis and herbology with Michael at workshops held throughout the country.

Lesley and Michael are available for consultations and acupuncture treatments at their clinic in Santa Cruz, Ca. Write or call: 208 Locust st., Santa Cruz, Ca. 95061; (408) 429-8066.

EAST WEST HERBAL CORRESPONDENCE COURSE

A comprehensive 36 lesson herbal correspondence course integrating principles of Western, Chinese and Ayurvedic herbalism. Students progress at their own pace with projects, questions and study guides which are reported on at the end of each lesson and submitted for approval.

The lessons include principles of balanced dietary therapy, traditional herbal diagnosis, making home preparations, identifying local herbs, a materia medica of well over 400 herbs from around the world, important traditional formulas used by master herbalists, including the most important Chinese and Ayurvedic formulas as well as possible Western equivalents.

Personal workshops are offered by Michael and Lesley at various intervals throughout the year and students are encouraged to attend for further studies. Students are also notified of other herbal gatherings and events that occur from time to time throughout the country.

Upon completion, students are given a certificate of completion signed by Michael and Lesley Tierra. Course work will be counted towards partial accreditation in the American Herbalist Guild, a professional herbalists organization.

For those who seek only an introduction to holistic herbal principles, there is also a shorter 12 lesson course. This is suitable for store owners and individuals involved in the marketing and sales of herbs.

For further information write East West Herbal Correspondence Course, Box 712W, Santa Cruz, Ca. 95061

PLANETHERB

NOW THERE IS A NEW WAY TO FIND THE RIGHT
HERBS WITH SPEED AND ACURRACY.

Planet-Herb is an herbal data base which includes over 448 Western and Chinese herbs and an editor for adding virtually unlimited numbers of herbs and information as needed.

With PLANETHERB you can have the memory of the World's herbal knowledge. 448 HERBS!!

CROSS-REFERENCING takes just seconds.

CHINESE herbs, conditions and properties included.

PROPERTY CATEGORIES can be searched as a whole.

CONTRA-INDICATIONS are entered with a keystroke.

You can learn to use PLANETHERB in just a few minutes! Built-in menus allow you to select search keywords without spelling them out.

Available in PC hard disk version, MAC and ST versions.

Write Steve Blake, SR1 Box 35, Haiku, Hi 96708